AF770575

The Pelvic Floor Handbook

A Guide to Understanding and Treating Pelvic Floor Disorders

Cassidy J. Parrish

Xspurts.com

A New Zealand Designed Product

Other Versions Available

Why limit yourself to just one format?

This book is now available in physical, digital, and audiobook options.

Choose the way you love to read and dive into the story today. You won't regret it!

Digital ISBN: 9781776848072
Physical ISBN: 9781776846986
Audio ISBN:

To obtain a different format of this book at a discounted price, please get in touch with us at:

http://isbn.xspurts.com/

Contents

Chapter One

Introduction to the Pelvic Floor

The pelvic floor is a complex network of muscles, ligaments, and connective tissue that forms a sling-like structure at the base of the pelvis. Its function is to support the organs in the pelvis, such as the bladder, uterus, and rectum, as well as to control the passage of urine and feces. Despite its important role in our bodily functions, the pelvic floor is often overlooked and neglected. Below we will delve into the pelvic floor and discuss its anatomy, function, and the common issue of pelvic floor dysfunction.

Anatomy of the Pelvic Floor

The pelvic floor is composed of several layers of muscles and tissues that work together to provide support and control. The first layer is the superficial layer, which consists of the bulbo-cavernosus, ischiocavernosus, and superficial transverse perineal muscles. The second layer is the intermediate layer, which is made up of the urethral and vaginal sphincters, as well as the deep transverse perineal muscle. Finally, the deep layer of the pelvic floor is comprised of the levator ani muscle, which includes the pubococcygeus, puborectalis, and iliococcygeus muscles.

Function of the Pelvic Floor

The pelvic floor has several crucial functions. First and foremost, it provides support for the organs in the pelvis, including the bladder, uterus, and rectum. This support prevents these organs from descending and bulging into the vaginal or rectal canal. Additionally, the pelvic floor plays a critical role in controlling the passage of urine and feces. The muscles of the pelvic floor work in conjunction with the urethral and anal sphincters to hold in urine and feces until it is time to go to the bathroom. Finally, the pelvic floor is involved in sexual function. During sexual activity, the muscles of the pelvic floor contract and relax, aiding in sexual arousal and orgasm.

Pelvic Floor Dysfunction

Pelvic floor dysfunction is a condition that affects both men and women and can cause a variety of symptoms, including urinary and fecal incontinence, chronic pelvic pain, painful intercourse, and constipation. The causes of pelvic floor dysfunction are varied and can include childbirth, surgery, aging, obesity, chronic coughing, and certain neurological conditions.

One common type of pelvic floor dysfunction is stress urinary incontinence (SUI). SUI occurs when the muscles of the pelvic floor are weak and can no longer support the bladder as well as they once did. This results in involuntary leakage of urine during activities such as coughing, sneezing, laughing, or lifting heavy objects. Another type of pelvic floor dysfunction is urge urinary incontinence. This occurs when the muscles of the bladder contract involuntarily, causing a sudden and intense need to urinate. People with urge urinary incontinence may experience leakage of urine before they can make it to the bathroom.

Treatment for Pelvic Floor Dysfunction

The treatment for pelvic floor dysfunction varies depending on the type and severity of the condition. In mild cases, lifestyle modifications such as pelvic floor exercises, dietary changes, and weight loss may be recommended. Pelvic floor exercises, also known as Kegels, involve contracting and relaxing the muscles of the pelvic floor to strengthen them. These exercises can be done anywhere and at any time, making them a convenient and effective way to improve pelvic floor function.

For more severe cases of pelvic floor dysfunction, more advanced treatment options may be necessary. These options can include medication, biofeedback, pelvic floor physical therapy, and even surgery. Medications may be used to relax the muscles of the bladder or to reduce inflammation and pain. Biofeedback involves using electronic sensors to monitor muscle activity in the pelvic floor and provide feedback on how to improve control of these muscles. This method helps individuals learn how to contract and relax their pelvic floor muscles more effectively, enhancing their strength and coordination.

Pelvic floor physical therapy is another crucial treatment avenue. This specialized form of physical therapy focuses on the rehabilitation of the pelvic floor muscles. A trained pelvic floor physical therapist can guide individuals through exercises tailored to their specific condition, helping to alleviate symptoms and improve quality of life. These therapists may also employ techniques such as manual therapy to release muscle tension and improve muscle function.

Surgery may be considered as a last resort for those who do not respond to other treatments. Surgical options vary depending on the specific type of pelvic floor dysfunction. For example, in cases of severe stress urinary incontinence, procedures that support the urethra or bladder neck, such as sling procedures, may be recommended.

Additionally, lifestyle and behavioral modifications play a vital role in managing and treating pelvic floor dysfunction. These may include bladder training to manage urge urinary incontinence, avoiding heavy lifting, and learning proper body mechanics to reduce strain on the pelvic floor.

Managing constipation through diet, hydration, and bowel management strategies can also alleviate pressure on the pelvic floor.

It's essential for individuals suffering from pelvic floor dysfunction to consult with a healthcare professional who can assess their condition and recommend a personalized treatment plan. With the right combination of treatments, many people with pelvic floor dysfunction can achieve significant improvement in their symptoms and quality of life.

Ultimately, the journey to recovery from pelvic floor dysfunction is a collaborative process that may involve various specialists, including urologists, gynecologists, physical therapists, and dietitians. By understanding the condition and actively participating in the treatment process, individuals can navigate their way towards better pelvic health.

What is a Pelvic Floor?

The pelvic floor is a group of muscles and tissues that form a supportive hammock-like structure at the bottom of the pelvis. This vital part of the body plays a significant role in the control of the bladder, bowels, and sexual function. However, many people are not familiar with the pelvic floor until they experience pelvic floor dysfunction. Below we will discuss what the pelvic floor is, its functions, and the causes and treatments for pelvic floor dysfunction.

Anatomy of the Pelvic Floor

The pelvic floor is made up of muscles, ligaments, and connective tissues that stretch across the bottom of the pelvis. The pelvic floor is comprised of three layers of muscles: the superficial layer, the intermediate layer, and the deep layer.

The superficial layer of the pelvic floor is composed of the bulbo-cavernosus, ischiocavernosus, and superficial transverse perineal muscles. These muscles are responsible for controlling the base of the penis or the clitoris.

The intermediate layer of the pelvic floor includes the urethral and vaginal sphincters and the deep transverse perineal muscle. The urethral sphincter helps control the flow of urine, while the vaginal sphincter helps control the flow of blood during menstruation.

The deep layer of the pelvic floor includes the levator ani muscle, which is made up of three separate muscles: the pubococcygeus, puborectalis, and iliococcygeus. These muscles work together to support the pelvic organs and control the anal sphincter.

Function of the Pelvic Floor

The pelvic floor muscles are responsible for several vital functions in the body, including providing support for the pelvic organs, controlling the bladder and bowel movements, and aiding in sexual function.

The pelvic organs, including the bladder, uterus, and rectum, are supported by the pelvic floor muscles. When these muscles weaken or become damaged, the pelvic organs can sag and bulge, leading to pelvic organ prolapse.

The pelvic floor muscles also help control the bladder and bowel movements. The muscles work together with the urinary and anal sphincters to hold urine and feces in until it is time to go to the bathroom.

Finally, the pelvic floor muscles are involved in sexual function. During sexual activity, the muscles contract and relax, contributing to sexual arousal and orgasm.

Pelvic Floor Dysfunction

Pelvic floor dysfunction is a term used to describe a range of conditions that affect the muscles, ligaments, and connective tissue in the pelvic floor. This condition affects both men and women, but it is more common in women, especially those who have given birth.

There are several types of pelvic floor dysfunction, including urinary incontinence, fecal incontinence, pelvic organ prolapse, and chronic pelvic pain.

Urinary incontinence is a condition where a person experiences involuntary leakage of urine. This condition can be caused by weak pelvic floor muscles or an overactive bladder.

Fecal incontinence is a condition where a person experiences involuntary leakage of feces. This condition can be caused by damage to the pelvic floor muscles or nerves.

Pelvic organ prolapse occurs when the pelvic organs, such as the bladder, uterus, or rectum, bulge into the vaginal canal due to weakened or damaged pelvic floor muscles.

Chronic pelvic pain is a condition where a person experiences pain in the pelvic region that lasts for more than six months. This condition can be caused by a variety of factors, including pelvic floor muscle dysfunction.

Treatment for Pelvic Floor Dysfunction

The treatment for pelvic floor dysfunction varies depending on the type and severity of the condition. In mild cases, lifestyle modifications such as pelvic floor exercises, dietary changes, and weight loss may be recommended. Pelvic floor exercises, also known as Kegels, involve contracting and relaxing the pelvic floor muscles. These exercises can help strengthen the muscles that support the bladder, uterus, and rectum, improving symptoms of urinary incontinence, fecal incontinence, and pelvic organ prolapse.

For those experiencing chronic pelvic pain, treatment may focus on managing pain through a combination of physical therapy, medication, and sometimes counseling to address any psychological components of chronic pain. Physical therapy can include specific exercises to stretch and strengthen the pelvic floor muscles, as well as manual therapy techniques to relieve muscle tension.

In addition to exercises, biofeedback therapy is another non-invasive treatment option for pelvic floor dysfunction. Biofeedback helps individuals gain better awareness and control of their pelvic floor muscles. Using special sensors, patients can see real-time feedback on a monitor, helping them understand how to properly contract and relax their pelvic floor muscles.

For individuals with severe or persistent symptoms, more advanced treatments may be necessary. These could include electrical stimulation to strengthen the pelvic floor muscles or surgery for cases of severe pelvic organ prolapse or when other treatments have failed to provide relief.

Lifestyle and dietary changes can also play a significant role in managing symptoms. For instance, avoiding foods and drinks that irritate the bladder can help reduce urinary incontinence. Similarly, maintaining a healthy weight and avoiding heavy lifting can relieve pressure on the pelvic floor and mitigate symptoms.

It's important for individuals experiencing symptoms of pelvic floor dysfunction to consult a healthcare professional for a proper diagnosis and personalized treatment plan. Healthcare providers may include gynecologists, urologists, colorectal surgeons, or physical therapists specializing in pelvic floor disorders.

Ultimately, the goal of treatment for pelvic floor dysfunction is to improve the individual's quality of life by reducing or eliminating symptoms. With the right combination of treatments, many people can achieve significant improvements and regain control over their pelvic health.

Importance of pelvic floor health

The pelvic floor is a crucial part of the body that is often overlooked until problems arise. It is made up of a group of muscles and tissues that form a supportive hammock-like structure at the bottom of the pelvis. The pelvic floor plays a vital role in supporting the bladder, bowel, and sexual function. Below we will discuss the importance of pelvic floor health and the consequences of pelvic floor dysfunction.

The Importance of Pelvic Floor Health

A healthy pelvic floor is essential for maintaining good quality of life. It is responsible for supporting the pelvic organs, controlling bowel and bladder function, and aiding in sexual function. A strong and healthy pelvic floor can help prevent pelvic organ prolapse, urinary and fecal incontinence, and chronic pelvic pain.

Pelvic organ prolapse occurs when the pelvic organs, such as the bladder, uterus, or rectum, bulge into the vaginal canal due to weakened or damaged pelvic floor muscles. This condition can lead to discomfort, pain, and difficulties with bowel and bladder function. In severe cases, surgery may be necessary to correct the prolapse.

Urinary and fecal incontinence are common problems associated with pelvic floor dysfunction. Urinary incontinence is a condition where a person experiences involuntary leakage of urine. This condition can be caused by weak pelvic floor muscles or an overactive bladder. Fecal incontinence is a condition where a person experiences involuntary leakage of feces. This condition can be caused by damage to the pelvic floor muscles or nerves.

Chronic pelvic pain is another problem that can result from pelvic floor dysfunction. This condition can be caused by a variety of factors, including pelvic floor muscle dysfunction. Chronic pelvic pain can significantly impact a person's quality of life and may require medical intervention.

Prevention and Treatment of Pelvic Floor Dysfunction

Preventing pelvic floor dysfunction involves maintaining a healthy lifestyle, including regular exercise, a balanced diet, and avoiding smoking. Pelvic floor exercises, also known as Kegels, are a great way to keep the pelvic floor muscles strong and healthy. These exercises involve contracting and relaxing the muscles that support the bladder, bowel, and uterus.

In cases of pelvic floor dysfunction, treatment varies depending on the type and severity of the condition. In mild cases, lifestyle modifications such as pelvic floor exercises, dietary changes, and weight loss may be recommended. In more severe cases, medications, physical therapy, or surgery may be necessary to correct the problem.

Physical therapy is often used to treat pelvic floor dysfunction. This therapy may involve biofeedback, which helps patients learn how to control their pelvic floor muscles, or electrical stimulation, which can help strengthen weak muscles.

Surgery may be necessary in severe cases of pelvic floor dysfunction, such as pelvic organ prolapse or urinary incontinence. There are several surgical options available, including sling procedures, bladder suspension, and colposuspension.

Functions of the pelvic floor

The pelvic floor is a group of muscles and tissues that form a supportive structure at the bottom of the pelvis. This structure plays a vital role in supporting the pelvic organs, controlling bowel and bladder function, and aiding in sexual function. Below we will discuss the functions of the pelvic floor and the consequences of pelvic floor dysfunction.

Functions of the Pelvic Floor

The pelvic floor muscles perform several essential functions in the body. These include:

Support for Pelvic Organs

The pelvic floor provides support for the pelvic organs, including the bladder, uterus, and rectum. The muscles and tissues of the pelvic floor act as a hammock-like structure, holding these organs in place. This support is critical for maintaining the proper functioning of these organs.

Control of Bowel Function

The pelvic floor muscles play a crucial role in bowel function. These muscles work with the anal sphincter to control the release of feces from the body. The muscles help to maintain continence and prevent involuntary leakage of feces.

Control of Bladder Function

The pelvic floor muscles also play a critical role in bladder function. These muscles work with the bladder to control the release of urine from the body. The muscles help to maintain continence and prevent involuntary leakage of urine.

Sexual Function

The pelvic floor muscles are involved in sexual function, particularly in women. These muscles help to support the vagina, clitoris, and uterus, and aid in achieving orgasm. A strong and healthy pelvic floor can improve sexual function and satisfaction.

Pelvic Floor Dysfunction

Pelvic floor dysfunction is a common problem that occurs when the muscles and tissues of the pelvic floor are weakened or damaged. This condition can lead to a variety of problems, including urinary and fecal incontinence, pelvic organ prolapse, and chronic pelvic pain.

Urinary incontinence is a condition where a person experiences involuntary leakage of urine. This condition can be caused by weak pelvic floor muscles or an overactive bladder. Fecal incontinence is a condition where a person experiences involuntary leakage of feces. This condition can be caused by damage to the pelvic floor muscles or nerves.

Pelvic organ prolapse occurs when the pelvic organs, such as the bladder, uterus, or rectum, bulge into the vaginal canal due to weakened or damaged pelvic floor muscles. This condition can lead to discomfort, pain, and difficulties with bowel and bladder function. In severe cases, surgery may be necessary to correct the prolapse.

Chronic pelvic pain is another problem that can result from pelvic floor dysfunction. This condition can be caused by a variety of factors, including pelvic floor muscle dysfunction. Chronic pelvic pain can significantly impact a person's quality of life and may require medical intervention.

Prevention and Treatment of Pelvic Floor Dysfunction

Preventing pelvic floor dysfunction involves maintaining a healthy lifestyle, including regular exercise, a balanced diet, and avoiding smoking. Pelvic floor exercises, also known as Kegels, are a great way to keep the pelvic floor muscles strong and healthy. These exercises involve contracting and relaxing the muscles that support the bladder, bowel, and uterus.

In cases of pelvic floor dysfunction, treatment varies depending on the type and severity of the condition. In mild cases, lifestyle modifications such as pelvic floor exercises, dietary changes, and weight loss may be recommended. In more severe cases, medications, physical therapy, or surgery may be necessary to correct the problem.

Physical therapy is often used to treat pelvic floor dysfunction. This therapy may involve biofeedback, which helps patients learn how to control their pelvic floor muscles, or electrical stimulation, which can help strengthen weak muscles.

Surgery may be necessary in severe cases of pelvic floor dysfunction, such as pelvic organ prolapse or urinary incontinence. There are several surgical options available, including sling procedures for urinary incontinence, which support the urethra to prevent leakage, and repair surgeries for pelvic organ prolapse, where the prolapsed organ is lifted back into its original position. These surgical interventions aim to restore the normal function and support of the pelvic floor.

Medications can also play a role in managing symptoms associated with pelvic floor dysfunction. For example, anticholinergic drugs can help reduce symptoms of an overactive bladder, while laxatives may be used to manage constipation related to pelvic floor dysfunction.

It is essential for individuals experiencing symptoms of pelvic floor dysfunction to seek medical advice. A healthcare provider can offer a thorough evaluation and recommend a personalized treatment plan based on the individual's specific condition and needs.

Education on pelvic health is also crucial. Awareness of the pelvic floor's functions and the importance of maintaining its health can lead to early detection and prevention of dysfunction. Resources such as workshops, support groups, and informational materials can provide valuable information and support to those affected by pelvic floor dysfunction.

In summary, the pelvic floor plays a crucial role in various bodily functions, and dysfunction can lead to significant physical and emotional challenges. However, with proper prevention strategies, early intervention, and appropriate treatment, individuals can manage or overcome pelvic floor dysfunction and maintain a good quality of life.

The anatomy of the pelvic floor

The pelvic floor is a group of muscles and tissues that form a supportive structure at the bottom of the pelvis. The anatomy of the pelvic floor is complex and includes several layers of muscles, ligaments, and nerves. Below we will discuss the anatomy of the pelvic floor and its relevance to pelvic floor dysfunction.

The Pelvic Floor Muscles

The pelvic floor muscles are a group of muscles that extend from the pubic bone to the tailbone. These muscles form a hammock-like structure that supports the pelvic organs and aids in bowel, bladder, and sexual function. The pelvic floor muscles are divided into three layers: the superficial layer, the middle layer, and the deep layer.

The superficial layer is composed of the bulbospongiosus, ischiocavernosus, and transverse perineal muscles. These muscles are responsible for supporting the perineum, the area between the anus and the genitals.

The middle layer is composed of the external anal sphincter and the urethral sphincter. These muscles are responsible for controlling the release of feces and urine.

The deep layer is composed of the levator ani muscles, which are further divided into the puborectalis, pubococcygeus, and iliococcygeus muscles. These muscles are responsible for supporting the pelvic organs and maintaining continence.

The Pelvic Floor Ligaments

The pelvic floor also includes several ligaments that help to support the pelvic organs. These ligaments include the pubocervical ligament, which supports the cervix and uterus in women, and the cardinal ligament, which supports the uterus and vagina.

The Pelvic Floor Nerves

The pelvic floor is innervated by several nerves, including the pudendal nerve, which provides sensation to the perineum and controls the external anal sphincter and urethral sphincter. The pelvic floor is also innervated by the sacral nerves, which control the internal anal sphincter and pelvic organs.

Pelvic Floor Dysfunction and Anatomy

Pelvic floor dysfunction occurs when the muscles, ligaments, or nerves of the pelvic floor are weakened or damaged. This can lead to a variety of problems, including urinary and fecal incontinence, pelvic organ prolapse, and chronic pelvic pain.

Urinary incontinence occurs when the pelvic floor muscles are unable to properly control the release of urine from the bladder. This can be caused by damage to the nerves or muscles of the pelvic floor. Fecal incontinence occurs when the muscles of the pelvic floor are unable to properly control the release of feces from the rectum.

Pelvic organ prolapse occurs when the muscles and ligaments of the pelvic floor are weakened, causing the pelvic organs to bulge into the vagina. This can lead to discomfort, pain, and difficulties with bowel and bladder function.

Chronic pelvic pain is another problem that can result from pelvic floor dysfunction. This condition can be caused by a variety of factors, including damage to the nerves or muscles of the pelvic floor.

Diagnosing Pelvic Floor Dysfunction

Diagnosing pelvic floor dysfunction typically involves a physical exam, which may include a pelvic exam, and tests to assess bladder and bowel function. In some cases, imaging studies, such as an MRI or ultrasound, may be necessary to evaluate the pelvic floor muscles and organs.

Treating Pelvic Floor Dysfunction

Treating pelvic floor dysfunction typically involves a combination of lifestyle modifications, pelvic floor exercises, and, in some cases, medication or surgery.

Pelvic floor exercises, also known as Kegels, involve contracting and relaxing the muscles of the pelvic floor. These exercises can help to strengthen the muscles and improve bladder and bowel control.

In cases of severe pelvic floor dysfunction, medication or surgery may be necessary to address underlying issues or to repair damaged tissues. Medications may be prescribed to manage symptoms such as urinary urgency or incontinence, while surgical options may include procedures to support or lift prolapsed organs, or to repair the muscles and ligaments of the pelvic floor.

In addition to exercises and medical interventions, physical therapy can be a critical component of treatment for pelvic floor dysfunction. Pelvic floor physical therapists specialize in evaluating and treating conditions related to the pelvic floor. They may use techniques such as manual therapy to relieve muscle tension, biofeedback to improve awareness and control of pelvic floor muscles, and education on proper pelvic floor function during everyday activities.

Lifestyle modifications can also play a significant role in managing and preventing pelvic floor dysfunction. These may include dietary changes to prevent constipation, weight management to reduce pressure on the pelvic floor, and avoidance of activities that strain the pelvic floor muscles, such as heavy lifting.

Ultimately, the goal of treating pelvic floor dysfunction is to restore normal function and alleviate symptoms, improving the individual's quality of life. A multidisciplinary approach, involving healthcare providers, physical therapists, and the patient's active participation in their treatment plan, is often most effective in achieving these goals.

Understanding the complex anatomy of the pelvic floor and its role in supporting pelvic organs and functions is essential for recognizing and addressing pelvic floor dysfunction. With proper diagnosis and treatment, many individuals can find relief from their symptoms and enjoy a healthier, more comfortable life.

The causes of pelvic floor dysfunction

Pelvic floor dysfunction refers to the inability of the muscles, ligaments, and connective tissues of the pelvic floor to function correctly. This can lead to a variety of symptoms such as urinary incontinence, fecal incontinence, chronic pelvic pain, and sexual dysfunction. While the causes of pelvic floor dysfunction can vary, it is often a result of a combination of factors that contribute to weakened or overactive pelvic floor muscles. Below we will explore the common causes of pelvic floor dysfunction and how they can impact overall pelvic floor health.

One of the leading causes of pelvic floor dysfunction is pregnancy and childbirth. The weight of the growing fetus can place pressure on the pelvic floor muscles, leading to weakness and stretching. This stretching can result in tears and damage to the muscles and connective tissues, which can lead to urinary and fecal incontinence. Additionally, the act of giving birth can further weaken these muscles, as the stretching and pressure can cause trauma to the pelvic floor. Women who have had multiple pregnancies or delivered large babies are at a higher risk of developing pelvic floor dysfunction.

Another common cause of pelvic floor dysfunction is age. As we age, our muscles naturally weaken, and this can include the pelvic floor muscles. Hormonal changes during menopause can also impact pelvic floor health. The reduction of estrogen levels can lead to a decrease in muscle tone, which can contribute to incontinence and pelvic organ prolapse. Men can also experience pelvic floor dysfunction as they age, as the prostate gland can enlarge and place pressure on the pelvic floor muscles, causing urinary incontinence.

Chronic constipation is another cause of pelvic floor dysfunction. Straining to pass hard stools can weaken the pelvic floor muscles and cause stretching and damage. Over time, this can lead to fecal incontinence and pelvic organ prolapse.

Pelvic surgeries such as a hysterectomy, prostatectomy, or bladder surgery can also contribute to pelvic floor dysfunction. During these surgeries, the pelvic floor muscles may be damaged, leading to urinary or fecal incontinence, pelvic pain, and sexual dysfunction.

In addition to the physical causes of pelvic floor dysfunction, lifestyle factors can also play a role. Being overweight can place added pressure on the pelvic floor muscles, leading to weakness and stretching. Chronic coughing can also impact pelvic floor health, as the repeated strain on the muscles can lead to weakness and incontinence. Smoking can also contribute to pelvic floor dysfunction, as it can reduce blood flow to the pelvic area and weaken the muscles.

Lastly, psychological factors such as stress and anxiety can also impact pelvic floor health. When we experience stress, our bodies release hormones that can cause muscle tension and tightness. This tension can impact the pelvic floor muscles and contribute to chronic pain and incontinence. Additionally, anxiety can lead to increased frequency and urgency of urination, which can further weaken the pelvic floor muscles.

Chapter Two

Common Pelvic Floor Disorders

The pelvic floor is an essential part of the human body that supports the bladder, uterus, and rectum. It is a group of muscles and connective tissues that form a hammock-like structure at the bottom of the pelvis. The pelvic floor is responsible for various functions, including maintaining continence, supporting the pelvic organs, and facilitating sexual function. However, many people experience problems with their pelvic floor, which can lead to a range of disorders.

One of the most common pelvic floor disorders is urinary incontinence. Urinary incontinence is the unintentional leakage of urine. It can be caused by weakened or damaged pelvic floor muscles, which can occur due to childbirth, surgery, aging, or other medical conditions. Urinary incontinence can significantly impact a person's quality of life, leading to embarrassment, social isolation, and decreased physical activity.

Another common pelvic floor disorder is fecal incontinence, which is the involuntary loss of bowel control. Like urinary incontinence, fecal incontinence can be caused by weakened or damaged pelvic floor muscles. It can also result from nerve damage, injury to the anal sphincter, or conditions such as inflammatory bowel disease. Fecal incontinence can be particularly distressing for individuals, causing embarrassment and anxiety.

Pelvic organ prolapse is another condition that affects the pelvic floor. Pelvic organ prolapse occurs when one or more pelvic organs, such as the uterus, bladder, or rectum, drop from their normal position and press against the vaginal wall. This can be caused by weakened or damaged pelvic floor muscles, as well as childbirth, menopause, chronic constipation, or heavy lifting. Pelvic organ prolapse can cause discomfort, pain during sex, and difficulty with urination or bowel movements.

Sexual dysfunction is another common pelvic floor disorder that can result from weakened pelvic floor muscles. This can lead to a range of problems, including reduced sensation during sex, difficulty achieving orgasm, and pain during intercourse.

In addition to these specific disorders, the pelvic floor can also be affected by chronic pain conditions. Pelvic pain, for example, is a chronic pain condition that affects the pelvic region. It can be caused by a variety of factors, including pelvic floor muscle dysfunction, nerve damage, endometriosis, or interstitial cystitis. Chronic pelvic pain can be difficult to manage, leading to significant physical and emotional distress.

While these are some of the most common pelvic floor disorders, there are many other conditions that can affect the pelvic floor. It is essential to recognize the signs and symptoms of these conditions and seek medical attention if you experience any concerning symptoms.

Urinary incontinence

Urinary incontinence is a condition that affects millions of people worldwide. It is a type of pelvic floor dysfunction that occurs when the muscles in the pelvic area responsible for controlling the bladder are weakened or damaged. Urinary incontinence can be a source of great embarrassment and discomfort for those who suffer from it, and it can significantly impact their quality of life.

There are different types of urinary incontinence, each with its unique set of symptoms and causes. The most common types of urinary incontinence include stress incontinence, urge incontinence, and mixed incontinence.

Stress incontinence is a type of urinary incontinence that occurs when physical exertion or pressure on the bladder leads to involuntary urine leakage. This can happen during activities such as laughing, sneezing, coughing, or lifting heavy objects. Stress incontinence is most common in women and is often caused by pregnancy, childbirth, or menopause.

Urge incontinence, also known as overactive bladder, is a type of urinary incontinence that occurs when there is an urgent and sudden need to urinate, and the bladder muscle contracts involuntarily, leading to urine leakage. This type of incontinence can be caused by a variety of factors, such as neurological disorders, bladder infections, or bladder irritants such as caffeine or alcohol.

Mixed incontinence is a combination of stress and urge incontinence. It is the most common type of urinary incontinence in older adults and is often associated with conditions such as diabetes, obesity, or chronic obstructive pulmonary disease (COPD).

Urinary incontinence can also be caused by certain medical conditions, such as an enlarged prostate gland in men or a pelvic organ prolapse in women. In some cases, medications or surgeries can cause urinary incontinence as a side effect.

There are several ways to manage and treat urinary incontinence, depending on the severity of the condition and the underlying causes. Some common treatments include pelvic floor muscle exercises, bladder training, medication, and surgery.

Pelvic floor muscle exercises, also known as Kegels, involve contracting and relaxing the muscles that control the bladder and bowel. This type of exercise can help to strengthen the pelvic floor muscles and improve bladder control.

Bladder training involves gradually increasing the time between bathroom breaks to train the bladder to hold more urine. This can be helpful for people with urge incontinence who have a sudden and frequent urge to urinate.

Medications can also be prescribed to help manage urinary incontinence. For example, anticholinergics can be used to relax the bladder muscles and reduce the urge to urinate, while alpha-blockers can be used to relax the muscles around the urethra and improve urine flow in men with an enlarged prostate gland.

In some cases, surgery may be necessary to treat urinary incontinence. For example, surgery can be performed to support the bladder or urethra and prevent urine leakage.

Fecal

incontinence

Fecal incontinence, also known as bowel incontinence, is the involuntary loss of control over the bowels, leading to the unintentional passage of fecal matter. This condition can be embarrassing, and can have a profound impact on an individual's quality of life, making it difficult to engage in social activities and leading to depression and anxiety.

Fecal incontinence is more common than many people realize, and affects individuals of all ages and both genders. The prevalence of fecal incontinence varies depending on the population studied, but it is estimated to affect between 2% and 15% of the general population, with higher rates among the elderly, those with neurological disorders, and those with a history of pelvic surgery.

There are many causes of fecal incontinence, and it often results from damage to the muscles or nerves in the anal sphincter or rectum. Common causes of fecal incontinence include:

Damage to the anal sphincter: The anal sphincter is a group of muscles that control the opening and closing of the anus. Damage to these muscles can occur during childbirth, as a result of pelvic surgery, or as a result of injury or trauma to the pelvic area.

Neurological disorders: Neurological disorders, such as multiple sclerosis or spinal cord injury, can cause nerve damage that affects the ability to control bowel movements.

Chronic diarrhea: Chronic diarrhea can cause irritation and inflammation of the rectum, leading to fecal incontinence.

Constipation: Chronic constipation can lead to the stretching of the rectum, weakening the muscles and leading to fecal incontinence.

Aging: As we age, the muscles in the pelvic floor can weaken, leading to fecal incontinence.

The symptoms of fecal incontinence can vary depending on the severity of the condition. Some individuals may experience only occasional leakage of small amounts of stool, while others may experience complete loss of control over bowel movements. Individuals with fecal incontinence may experience anxiety, depression, and social isolation, which can further exacerbate the condition.

There are a number of treatments available for fecal incontinence, depending on the cause and severity of the condition. Treatment options may include dietary changes, medications, pelvic floor exercises, biofeedback therapy, and surgery.

Dietary changes: For individuals with fecal incontinence caused by chronic diarrhea or constipation, dietary changes may be effective. A high-fiber diet can help regulate bowel movements and prevent diarrhea or constipation.

Medications: Medications such as loperamide or bulking agents can help to control diarrhea and reduce the frequency of bowel movements, while laxatives or stool softeners can help to prevent constipation.

Pelvic floor exercises: Pelvic floor exercises, also known as Kegel exercises, can help to strengthen the muscles of the pelvic floor, improving control over bowel movements.

Biofeedback therapy: Biofeedback therapy uses electronic sensors to measure muscle contractions and provide feedback to the patient. This can help individuals with fecal incontinence to learn how to control their pelvic muscles and improve their bowel control.

Surgery: In severe cases, surgery may be necessary to repair damage to the anal sphincter or rectum. Surgery may also be recommended for individuals with neurological disorders that are affecting bowel control.

Pelvic organ prolapse

Pelvic organ prolapse (POP) is a common pelvic floor disorder that affects millions of women worldwide. It occurs when the pelvic organs, such as the uterus, bladder, or rectum, protrude or descend into the vaginal canal due to weakened pelvic floor muscles and ligaments. Below we will explore the causes, symptoms, diagnosis, and treatment options for pelvic organ prolapse.

Causes of Pelvic Organ Prolapse

There are several risk factors that contribute to the development of pelvic organ prolapse. These include age, pregnancy and childbirth, menopause, chronic coughing, obesity, and chronic constipation. Aging and hormonal changes that occur during menopause can cause weakening and thinning of pelvic floor muscles and ligaments. Pregnancy and childbirth can cause stretching and tearing of the pelvic floor muscles, leading to weakness and prolapse of the pelvic organs.

Symptoms of Pelvic Organ Prolapse

The symptoms of pelvic organ prolapse depend on the degree of organ prolapse and which organs are affected. Some women may not experience any symptoms, while others may have symptoms that affect their quality of life. Common symptoms of pelvic organ prolapse include:

A feeling of heaviness or pressure in the pelvic area

A bulging or protrusion from the vaginal opening

Difficulty urinating or defecating

Urinary incontinence or leaking urine during physical activity

Pain or discomfort during sexual intercourse

Diagnosis of Pelvic Organ Prolapse

Pelvic organ prolapse is diagnosed through a pelvic exam, where a doctor or gynecologist checks for signs of organ prolapse by looking for bulges in the vaginal canal. They may also perform imaging tests, such as a pelvic ultrasound, to assess the degree of prolapse and determine the organs affected.

Treatment of Pelvic Organ Prolapse

The treatment of pelvic organ prolapse depends on the severity of the prolapse, the organs affected, and the impact on the patient's quality of life. Treatment options include:

Pelvic floor exercises - These exercises, also known as Kegels, can help strengthen the pelvic floor muscles and improve symptoms of prolapse.

Pessary - A pessary is a device that is inserted into the vagina to support the pelvic organs and prevent prolapse.

Surgery - In severe cases of pelvic organ prolapse, surgery may be necessary to repair the weakened pelvic floor muscles and ligaments. Surgical options include vaginal surgery, abdominal surgery, or laparoscopic surgery.

Prevention of Pelvic Organ Prolapse

While some risk factors for pelvic organ prolapse are beyond our control, there are steps we can take to reduce our risk of developing this condition. These include:

Regular exercise - Physical activity can help maintain healthy pelvic floor muscles.

Maintain a healthy weight - Excess weight can put additional pressure on the pelvic floor muscles, leading to weakening and prolapse.

Avoid heavy lifting - Lifting heavy objects can cause strain on the pelvic floor muscles and increase the risk of prolapse.

Quit smoking - Smoking can contribute to chronic coughing, which can weaken the pelvic floor muscles.

Pain during intercourse

Pain during intercourse, also known as dyspareunia, is a common condition that affects many individuals, especially women. It is often associated with pelvic floor dysfunction, a condition that affects the muscles, ligaments, and connective tissue in the pelvic region. Below we will explore the causes, symptoms, and treatment options for pain during intercourse.

The pelvic floor muscles play a crucial role in sexual function. These muscles support the pelvic organs, including the bladder, uterus, and rectum. They also control the opening and closing of the vagina, which is essential for sexual intercourse. When the pelvic floor muscles are weak or damaged, they can cause pain during intercourse.

There are several factors that can contribute to pelvic floor dysfunction and pain during intercourse. One of the most common causes is childbirth. During childbirth, the pelvic floor muscles can become overstretched or torn, which can lead to weakness and dysfunction. Other factors that can contribute to pelvic floor dysfunction include aging, obesity, chronic constipation, and certain medical conditions such as endometriosis and pelvic inflammatory disease.

The symptoms of pain during intercourse can vary from person to person. Some individuals may experience a sharp or burning pain during penetration, while others may experience a deep ache or pressure in the pelvic region. In some cases, pain may occur only during certain positions or movements, such as deep penetration. Additionally, pain during intercourse can lead to anxiety and a decreased desire for sexual activity, which can further exacerbate the problem.

Treatment for pain during intercourse typically involves addressing the underlying cause of pelvic floor dysfunction. In some cases, pelvic floor exercises, also known as Kegel exercises, may be recommended to strengthen the pelvic floor muscles. These exercises involve contracting and relaxing the pelvic floor muscles, which can help improve muscle tone and reduce pain during intercourse.

Other treatments for pain during intercourse may include the use of vaginal dilators, which can help stretch and relax the vaginal muscles. Additionally, topical treatments such as lidocaine cream may be used to numb the area and reduce pain during intercourse. In some cases, surgery may be necessary to repair damaged pelvic floor muscles or correct other underlying medical conditions.

It is important to seek medical attention if you experience pain during intercourse. Your healthcare provider can help identify the underlying cause of your symptoms and recommend appropriate treatment options. Additionally, your healthcare provider may refer you to a pelvic floor physical therapist who can provide specialized care for pelvic floor dysfunction.

Pain in the pelvic area

The pelvic floor muscles are a complex system of muscles, ligaments, and tissues that form a supportive base for the pelvic organs. They play an essential role in a variety of bodily functions, including bladder and bowel control, sexual function, and overall stability of the pelvic region. However, pelvic floor dysfunction can lead to a variety of symptoms, including pain in the pelvic area.

Pelvic pain is a common symptom associated with pelvic floor dysfunction. It can manifest in a variety of ways, including sharp or dull pain, pressure, or discomfort in the pelvic region. The pain can be constant or intermittent, and it may worsen during certain activities, such as sexual intercourse, bowel movements, or prolonged periods of sitting or standing.

Pelvic pain can be caused by a variety of factors related to pelvic floor dysfunction. For example, hypertonic pelvic floor muscles, or muscles that are constantly contracted or tense, can cause pain and discomfort. Conversely, weak or underactive pelvic floor muscles can lead to instability in the pelvic region, which can cause pain and discomfort as well.

Another common cause of pelvic pain is pelvic organ prolapse, which occurs when one or more of the pelvic organs, such as the bladder or uterus, drop down into the vaginal canal due to weakened pelvic floor muscles. This can cause pressure and pain in the pelvic region, particularly during activities such as standing or walking.

Pain during sexual intercourse is another symptom commonly associated with pelvic floor dysfunction. Dyspareunia, or painful intercourse, can be caused by a variety of factors related to pelvic floor dysfunction, including hypertonic or weak pelvic floor muscles, scar tissue, or nerve damage.

In some cases, pelvic pain may be caused by nerve entrapment or compression, particularly in the pudendal nerve, which runs through the pelvic region and controls sensation in the genital area. Nerve entrapment can cause pain, numbness, or tingling in the pelvic region, as well as sexual dysfunction and bladder or bowel control problems.

Treatment for pelvic pain related to pelvic floor dysfunction depends on the underlying cause. In some cases, lifestyle changes such as exercise and weight management can be effective in reducing symptoms. Physical therapy, including pelvic floor muscle training and relaxation techniques, may also be recommended to help improve muscle function and reduce pain.

In cases where nerve entrapment or compression is the cause of pelvic pain, nerve blocks or surgical intervention may be necessary. In rare cases, surgery may be necessary to repair or reinforce weakened pelvic floor muscles, particularly in cases of pelvic organ prolapse.

Urinary urgency and frequency

Urinary urgency and frequency are common symptoms of pelvic floor dysfunction, a condition that affects many individuals, especially women. The pelvic floor is a complex system of muscles, ligaments, and nerves that support the pelvic organs, including the bladder, uterus, and rectum. Dysfunction of the pelvic floor can cause various urinary problems, such as urinary incontinence, urinary urgency, and frequency.

Urinary urgency is the sudden, strong urge to urinate that cannot be delayed. This condition can be highly disruptive to a person's life, causing them to interrupt their daily activities frequently to use the bathroom. It can also lead to urinary incontinence, where a person involuntarily leaks urine. Urinary frequency, on the other hand, is the need to urinate more frequently than usual, often more than eight times per day.

Pelvic floor dysfunction can be caused by various factors, such as pregnancy, childbirth, menopause, obesity, chronic coughing, and aging. Pregnancy and childbirth can cause stretching and weakening of the pelvic floor muscles, leading to urinary problems. Menopause can cause a decrease in estrogen levels, which can result in the thinning and weakening of the pelvic floor muscles. Chronic coughing can also weaken the pelvic floor muscles, as can obesity, which puts extra pressure on the pelvic floor.

One type of pelvic floor dysfunction that can cause urinary urgency and frequency is overactive bladder syndrome (OAB). OAB is a condition that causes a sudden and uncontrollable urge to urinate, often resulting in urinary incontinence. It is caused by the involuntary contraction of the detrusor muscle in the bladder, which causes the bladder to empty without warning. OAB can also be caused by nerve damage, neurological conditions, or urinary tract infections.

Another condition that can cause urinary urgency and frequency is interstitial cystitis (IC). IC is a chronic bladder condition that causes pain and pressure in the bladder and pelvic region, as well as frequent urination. The cause of IC is unknown, but it is believed to be related to inflammation of the bladder lining or an autoimmune response.

Treatment for urinary urgency and frequency caused by pelvic floor dysfunction depends on the underlying cause. One effective treatment is pelvic floor physical therapy, which involves exercises to strengthen and retrain the pelvic floor muscles. Biofeedback, electrical stimulation, and vaginal weights can also be used to help improve muscle control and coordination.

In addition to physical therapy, lifestyle changes can also help improve urinary symptoms caused by pelvic floor dysfunction. These changes may include dietary modifications, such as avoiding caffeine and alcohol, and increasing water intake. Bladder retraining, which involves gradually increasing the time between bathroom trips, can also be effective in improving urinary frequency and urgency.

In some cases, medication may be prescribed to help manage urinary urgency and frequency caused by pelvic floor dysfunction. These medications may include anticholinergics or beta-3 agonists, which work to relax the bladder muscles and reduce the urge to urinate. In severe cases, surgery may be recommended to correct pelvic floor dysfunction, such as a sling procedure to support the bladder or urethra.

Constipation

The pelvic floor is a complex network of muscles, ligaments, and connective tissues that act as a support structure for the organs located in the pelvis. These organs include the bladder, uterus, and rectum. The pelvic floor plays an essential role in many bodily functions, such as urination, bowel movements, and sexual intercourse. Dysfunction of the pelvic floor can cause a variety of problems, including constipation.

Constipation is a common condition that affects many people worldwide. It is characterized by difficulty passing stools, infrequent bowel movements, and hard stools. Constipation can occur for many reasons, including diet, lifestyle, and medication use. However, one often overlooked cause of constipation is pelvic floor dysfunction.

The pelvic floor muscles are responsible for controlling the opening and closing of the rectum. If these muscles are weak or not functioning correctly, they may not be able to contract properly, leading to difficulty passing stools. Additionally, if the pelvic floor muscles are too tight, they may not be able to relax enough to allow stool to pass through easily.

There are several types of pelvic floor dysfunction that can contribute to constipation. One common condition is pelvic floor muscle dysfunction. This occurs when the muscles of the pelvic floor are weak, tight, or both. It can be caused by factors such as pregnancy, childbirth, menopause, aging, surgery, or trauma. Symptoms of pelvic floor muscle dysfunction include difficulty passing stools, straining, and a feeling of incomplete emptying of the bowels.

Another type of pelvic floor dysfunction that can cause constipation is rectal prolapse. This occurs when the rectum falls down into the anal canal, making it difficult to pass stools. Symptoms of rectal prolapse include constipation, straining, and a feeling of pressure in the rectum.

Pelvic organ prolapse is another condition that can contribute to constipation. This occurs when one or more of the pelvic organs, such as the bladder, uterus, or rectum, drop down from their normal position and push against the vaginal wall. This can cause a feeling of pressure and discomfort in the pelvic area, making it difficult to pass stools.

Urinary incontinence is also often associated with pelvic floor dysfunction and constipation. Urinary incontinence occurs when there is a loss of bladder control, leading to an involuntary leakage of urine. This condition can occur due to weakened pelvic floor muscles or nerve damage. It can cause constipation by making it difficult to strain properly during bowel movements.

Diagnosis of pelvic floor dysfunction and constipation usually involves a physical examination by a healthcare provider, along with imaging studies such as ultrasound or magnetic resonance imaging (MRI). Treatment options may include pelvic floor exercises to strengthen or relax the muscles, medication to help with constipation, and in severe cases, surgery.

Other disorders

The pelvic floor is a complex network of muscles, ligaments, and tissues that support the pelvic organs, including the bladder, uterus, and rectum. Pelvic floor dysfunction (PFD) occurs when these muscles and tissues become weak or damaged, leading to a range of symptoms and disorders. In addition to the well-known conditions such as urinary incontinence and pelvic organ prolapse, PFD can also cause a variety of other disorders.

One such disorder is chronic pelvic pain (CPP). CPP is defined as non-cyclical pain that lasts for more than six months and is localized to the pelvic region. It can be caused by a range of factors, including PFD, endometriosis, irritable bowel syndrome, and interstitial cystitis. Symptoms of CPP can include pain during sexual intercourse, difficulty urinating, and constipation.

Another condition associated with PFD is vulvodynia, which is characterized by chronic pain and discomfort in the vulva area. The exact cause of vulvodynia is not known, but it is believed to be related to nerve damage, PFD, or hormonal imbalances. Symptoms can include burning, itching, and pain during sex.

Interstitial cystitis (IC) is a condition characterized by chronic inflammation of the bladder wall, resulting in pelvic pain and urinary urgency and frequency. IC is more common in women than in men, and PFD can be a contributing factor to the development of this disorder.

Pelvic floor dysfunction can also contribute to chronic constipation. The pelvic floor muscles are essential for defecation, and weak or damaged muscles can lead to difficulty passing stool. Symptoms of chronic constipation can include infrequent bowel movements, hard or lumpy stools, and a feeling of incomplete evacuation.

PFD can also cause a range of sexual dysfunctions, including erectile dysfunction (ED) in men and pain during intercourse in women. In men, PFD can interfere with blood flow to the penis, leading to difficulty achieving or maintaining an erection. In women, PFD can cause pain during penetration, leading to avoidance of sexual activity.

In addition to these conditions, PFD can also cause bladder pain syndrome, chronic prostatitis/chronic pelvic pain syndrome in men, and levator ani syndrome, which is characterized by chronic pain in the pelvic floor muscles. All of these conditions can significantly impact an individual's quality of life and require proper diagnosis and treatment.

Diagnosis of PFD typically involves a physical examination by a healthcare provider, who will assess the strength and function of the pelvic floor muscles. Additional diagnostic tests may include a pelvic ultrasound or MRI, urodynamic testing to measure bladder function, or a cystoscopy to examine the bladder wall.

Treatment for PFD depends on the specific condition and its underlying causes. Physical therapy, including pelvic floor muscle exercises, is often recommended as a first-line treatment for PFD. In addition, medications such as muscle relaxants, pain relievers, and antispasmodics may be prescribed to manage symptoms. In some cases, surgery may be necessary to repair or reinforce damaged pelvic floor muscles.

Chapter Three

Causes of Pelvic Floor Disorders

The pelvic floor is a group of muscles, ligaments, and connective tissue that form a sling-like structure at the base of the pelvis, supporting the bladder, uterus, rectum, and other pelvic organs. Pelvic floor disorders (PFDs) refer to a range of conditions caused by weakness or dysfunction of these muscles, leading to a variety of uncomfortable symptoms. Below we will explore the various causes of pelvic floor disorders.

Pregnancy and childbirth: PFDs are more common among women than men, and pregnancy and childbirth are among the primary reasons. During pregnancy, the weight of the growing uterus can put pressure on the pelvic floor muscles, leading to weakness or damage. Childbirth, especially vaginal delivery, can cause trauma to the pelvic floor muscles and nerves, resulting in conditions such as urinary incontinence and pelvic organ prolapse.

Aging: Aging can weaken the pelvic floor muscles and decrease their ability to support the pelvic organs. Hormonal changes during menopause can also contribute to the weakening of these muscles.

Obesity: Being overweight or obese can put excessive pressure on the pelvic floor muscles, leading to weakness or damage over time.

Chronic constipation: Straining to have a bowel movement can weaken the pelvic floor muscles over time, leading to conditions such as rectal prolapse and fecal incontinence.

Chronic coughing: Chronic coughing, such as that caused by smoking or respiratory conditions like chronic obstructive pulmonary disease (COPD), can put stress on the pelvic floor muscles and lead to their weakening or damage.

Genetics: Some people may be genetically predisposed to developing pelvic floor disorders. For example, a family history of connective tissue disorders can increase the risk of developing conditions such as pelvic organ prolapse.

Neurological conditions: Certain neurological conditions, such as multiple sclerosis, can affect the nerves that control the pelvic floor muscles, leading to PFDs.

Surgery: Pelvic surgery, especially procedures involving the reproductive organs or the rectum, can damage the pelvic floor muscles and lead to PFDs.

Trauma: Trauma to the pelvic area, such as that caused by a fall or accident, can damage the pelvic floor muscles and nerves, leading to PFDs.

Lifestyle factors: Certain lifestyle factors, such as heavy lifting or high-impact exercise, can put stress on the pelvic floor muscles and lead to their weakening over time.

Pregnancy and childbirth

Pregnancy and childbirth are important milestones in a woman's life, but they can also lead to changes in the body, including the pelvic floor. The pelvic floor is a group of muscles and connective tissue that supports the bladder, uterus, and rectum. During pregnancy and childbirth, the pelvic floor can become weakened or damaged, leading to pelvic floor dysfunction. Below we will discuss the effects of pregnancy and childbirth on the pelvic floor and the resulting pelvic floor disorders.

During pregnancy, hormonal changes can lead to increased blood flow and fluid retention in the pelvic area. This can cause the pelvic floor muscles to stretch and weaken, leading to urinary incontinence, fecal incontinence, and pelvic organ prolapse. As the fetus grows, it puts pressure on the pelvic floor, which can further weaken the muscles and cause additional problems.

Childbirth is also a significant contributor to pelvic floor dysfunction. During vaginal delivery, the baby's head passes through the pelvic floor muscles, which can cause them to stretch and tear. This can lead to urinary incontinence, fecal incontinence, and pelvic organ prolapse. The risk of pelvic floor damage during childbirth is higher for women who have had multiple births, had a large baby, or had a long labor.

It is important to note that not all women who give birth will experience pelvic floor dysfunction, and some women who have never given birth may also experience pelvic floor disorders. Other factors that can contribute to pelvic floor dysfunction include obesity, chronic coughing, and aging.

There are steps that women can take to reduce the risk of pelvic floor dysfunction during and after pregnancy. One of the most effective ways to prevent pelvic floor damage during childbirth is to do pelvic floor exercises, also known as Kegels, before and during pregnancy. These exercises involve squeezing and relaxing the pelvic floor muscles and can help strengthen them, reducing the risk of damage during delivery.

In addition to pelvic floor exercises, women can also take other steps to support the pelvic floor during and after pregnancy. Maintaining a healthy weight and staying active can help reduce the strain on the pelvic floor muscles. Avoiding heavy lifting and constipation can also help reduce the risk of pelvic floor damage.

If a woman does experience pelvic floor dysfunction during or after pregnancy, there are treatments available. Pelvic floor physical therapy can help strengthen the muscles and improve bladder and bowel control. In some cases, surgery may be necessary to repair the pelvic floor and correct the underlying issue.

Aging

The aging process is a natural part of life that affects all areas of the body, including the pelvic floor. The pelvic floor is a group of muscles, ligaments, and tissues that support the bladder, uterus, and rectum. As we age, changes occur in the pelvic floor that can lead to pelvic floor dysfunction. Below we will discuss the effects of aging on the pelvic floor and how it can contribute to pelvic floor disorders.

As we age, the muscles in the pelvic floor weaken and lose their elasticity. This can result in a variety of pelvic floor disorders, including urinary incontinence, fecal incontinence, and pelvic organ prolapse. The weakening of the pelvic floor muscles can be caused by a variety of factors, including hormonal changes, chronic medical conditions, and lifestyle factors such as smoking and obesity.

One of the most significant contributors to pelvic floor dysfunction in aging women is menopause. Menopause causes a decrease in estrogen levels, which can lead to changes in the vaginal tissue and pelvic floor muscles. The decrease in estrogen can cause the tissues to become thinner, less elastic, and less able to withstand pressure, leading to pelvic floor disorders such as urinary incontinence and pelvic organ prolapse.

Chronic medical conditions, such as obesity, diabetes, and hypertension, can also contribute to pelvic floor dysfunction in aging individuals. Obesity can put pressure on the pelvic floor muscles and weaken them over time. Diabetes can lead to nerve damage and affect the function of the pelvic floor muscles, leading to incontinence and prolapse. Hypertension can cause damage to the blood vessels that supply the pelvic floor muscles, leading to weakness and dysfunction.

Lifestyle factors such as smoking and a sedentary lifestyle can also contribute to pelvic floor dysfunction in aging individuals. Smoking can cause damage to the blood vessels that supply the pelvic floor muscles, leading to weakness and dysfunction. A sedentary lifestyle can lead to weakened muscles throughout the body, including the pelvic floor muscles.

In addition to the physical changes that occur in the pelvic floor with aging, psychological factors can also contribute to pelvic floor dysfunction. Aging individuals may experience anxiety, depression, and stress, which can affect their ability to control their bladder and bowel movements. These psychological factors can also lead to changes in the pelvic floor muscles, making them weaker and more susceptible to dysfunction.

There are several ways to prevent and manage pelvic floor dysfunction in aging individuals. Pelvic floor exercises, also known as Kegel exercises, can help strengthen the muscles in the pelvic floor and improve their elasticity. Maintaining a healthy weight, quitting smoking, and staying physically active can also help prevent pelvic floor dysfunction.

For individuals who are experiencing pelvic floor dysfunction, there are several treatment options available. In some cases, lifestyle changes such as those mentioned above can be enough to improve symptoms. In other cases, medications such as hormone therapy or nerve stimulators may be prescribed. For more severe cases, surgery may be required to correct pelvic organ prolapse or other pelvic floor disorders.

Obesity

Obesity is a growing problem worldwide, and it has been linked to several health issues, including pelvic floor dysfunction. Pelvic floor dysfunction refers to a range of conditions that affect the muscles, ligaments, and tissues that support the pelvic organs, including the bladder, uterus, and rectum. Below we will explore the link between obesity and pelvic floor dysfunction, examining how excess weight can contribute to the development of these conditions and what can be done to prevent or manage them.

One of the main ways in which obesity contributes to pelvic floor dysfunction is through the increased pressure it places on the pelvic organs. Excess weight can put pressure on the pelvic floor muscles, causing them to weaken over time. This can lead to a range of symptoms, including incontinence, pelvic pain, and prolapse. Furthermore, obesity is also linked to the development of conditions such as diabetes and heart disease, which can further contribute to pelvic floor dysfunction.

Studies have shown that women who are obese are more likely to experience pelvic floor dysfunction than those who are of a healthy weight. In particular, obesity has been linked to an increased risk of urinary incontinence, which is a common symptom of pelvic floor dysfunction. This is because the excess weight puts pressure on the bladder and urethra, making it more difficult to control urine flow. Similarly, obesity has also been linked to an increased risk of fecal incontinence, which is the inability to control bowel movements. This is because excess weight can put pressure on the rectum, making it more difficult to control the muscles that regulate bowel movements.

In addition to urinary and fecal incontinence, obesity is also linked to an increased risk of pelvic organ prolapse. This occurs when the pelvic organs, such as the uterus, bladder, or rectum, slip out of place and bulge into the vagina. The weakened pelvic floor muscles in obese women make them more susceptible to prolapse. Furthermore, obesity is also linked to sexual dysfunction, including pain during intercourse, which can be caused by pelvic floor dysfunction.

Fortunately, there are steps that can be taken to prevent or manage pelvic floor dysfunction in obese women. One of the most important steps is weight loss. Losing weight can reduce the pressure on the pelvic organs, which can help to strengthen the pelvic floor muscles over time. This, in turn, can reduce the risk of incontinence, prolapse, and other symptoms of pelvic floor dysfunction.

In addition to weight loss, pelvic floor exercises can also be effective in preventing and managing pelvic floor dysfunction. These exercises involve squeezing and relaxing the muscles of the pelvic floor, which can help to strengthen them over time. This, in turn, can improve bladder and bowel control, reduce prolapse symptoms, and even improve sexual function.

Finally, it is important for women who are obese to seek medical attention if they are experiencing symptoms of pelvic floor dysfunction. There are a range of treatment options available, including medication, surgery, and other interventions that can help to manage symptoms and improve quality of life.

Menopause

Menopause is a natural biological process that marks the end of a woman's reproductive years. During this time, the body undergoes many changes due to a decrease in estrogen production. These changes can affect a woman's overall health, including the health of her pelvic floor. Below we will discuss menopause and its connection to pelvic floor dysfunction.

Pelvic floor dysfunction is a condition that affects many women, particularly as they age. It refers to the inability of the pelvic floor muscles to function correctly, leading to symptoms such as urinary and fecal incontinence, pelvic pain, and sexual dysfunction. Menopause can exacerbate these symptoms and increase the risk of developing pelvic floor disorders.

One of the most significant changes that occur during menopause is a decrease in estrogen levels. Estrogen is a hormone that helps keep the pelvic floor healthy by maintaining the strength and elasticity of the tissues. As estrogen levels decline, the pelvic floor muscles can become weaker and less able to support the pelvic organs.

This weakened support can lead to pelvic organ prolapse, a condition in which one or more pelvic organs, such as the uterus or bladder, drop down and press against the vaginal wall. Pelvic organ prolapse can cause discomfort, pain during intercourse, and urinary incontinence.

Another common symptom of menopause is vaginal dryness. This occurs due to a decrease in the production of vaginal lubrication, which can cause discomfort during sexual activity. This discomfort can lead to a reduction in sexual activity and arousal, which can further weaken the pelvic floor muscles.

Additionally, menopause can lead to changes in the urinary tract, such as urinary urgency and frequency. These symptoms can be caused by a loss of bladder elasticity and capacity, which can occur due to a decrease in estrogen levels. When the bladder cannot hold as much urine as before, it can lead to more frequent trips to the bathroom and even urinary incontinence.

The risk of developing pelvic floor disorders also increases with age. As women get older, their pelvic floor muscles naturally weaken, making them more susceptible to conditions such as urinary and fecal incontinence, pelvic organ prolapse, and pelvic pain.

However, there are ways to manage the symptoms of pelvic floor dysfunction during menopause. One option is hormone replacement therapy (HRT), which involves taking estrogen supplements to maintain healthy estrogen levels. HRT can help relieve symptoms such as vaginal dryness and urinary incontinence and may even help prevent pelvic organ prolapse.

Another option is pelvic floor exercises, such as Kegels. These exercises involve contracting and relaxing the pelvic floor muscles to help strengthen them. Regular pelvic floor exercises can help prevent and manage symptoms of pelvic floor dysfunction.

Hysterectomy

Hysterectomy is a surgical procedure where a woman's uterus is removed. This is often done to treat certain medical conditions, such as uterine fibroids, endometriosis, or cancer of the uterus or cervix. Hysterectomy is a common procedure in the United States, with approximately 600,000 procedures performed annually. While it can be a life-saving procedure for some women, it can also result in pelvic floor dysfunction, which can cause a range of symptoms.

Pelvic floor dysfunction is a common condition that affects many women after a hysterectomy. This occurs when the muscles and connective tissue that support the pelvic organs become weakened or damaged, resulting in a range of symptoms. These symptoms can include urinary incontinence, fecal incontinence, pelvic pain, and pain during sex.

There are several factors that can contribute to pelvic floor dysfunction after a hysterectomy. One of the primary causes is damage to the pelvic nerves during the surgery. These nerves play an important role in controlling the muscles of the pelvic floor, and any damage can result in weakened or dysfunctional pelvic muscles. Additionally, the surgery itself can result in damage to the muscles and connective tissues that support the pelvic organs, leading to pelvic floor dysfunction.

Another factor that can contribute to pelvic floor dysfunction after a hysterectomy is hormonal changes. The removal of the uterus can cause changes in hormone levels, which can in turn affect the strength and tone of the pelvic floor muscles. Additionally, the hormonal changes associated with menopause, which often occur around the same time as a hysterectomy, can further contribute to pelvic floor dysfunction.

There are several steps that women can take to reduce their risk of developing pelvic floor dysfunction after a hysterectomy. One of the most important is to engage in pelvic floor exercises, also known as Kegel exercises, both before and after the surgery. These exercises involve contracting and relaxing the muscles of the pelvic floor, which can help to strengthen them and improve their function. Women can also work with a physical therapist to develop a customized exercise program that can help to address any specific pelvic floor issues they may be experiencing.

In addition to exercise, women can take steps to maintain a healthy weight, which can help to reduce the strain on the pelvic floor muscles. This can involve eating a healthy diet, engaging in regular physical activity, and managing any underlying medical conditions, such as diabetes or high blood pressure.

For women who do develop pelvic floor dysfunction after a hysterectomy, there are several treatment options available. These can include medications, such as muscle relaxants or hormone replacement therapy, as well as surgical procedures to repair or reconstruct the pelvic floor muscles. Additionally, many women find relief through non-surgical treatments, such as pelvic floor physical therapy or biofeedback.

Chronic coughing

Chronic coughing is a condition that can have a significant impact on a person's quality of life. It is defined as a cough that lasts for more than 8 weeks, and it can be caused by a variety of factors, such as allergies, asthma, or chronic obstructive pulmonary disease (COPD). However, chronic coughing can also lead to the development of pelvic floor dysfunction, which is a condition that affects the muscles, ligaments, and tissues that support the pelvic organs.

Pelvic floor dysfunction is a broad term that encompasses a range of conditions, including urinary incontinence, fecal incontinence, pelvic organ prolapse, pain during intercourse, and more. The pelvic floor is a complex system of muscles, ligaments, and tissues that work together to support the pelvic organs, including the bladder, uterus, and rectum. When the pelvic floor becomes weak or damaged, it can lead to a variety of problems, including those related to urinary and bowel function, sexual function, and overall quality of life.

One of the factors that can contribute to the development of pelvic floor dysfunction is chronic coughing. When a person coughs, the abdominal muscles contract forcefully, which can put pressure on the pelvic floor. Over time, this repeated pressure can lead to damage to the pelvic floor muscles and tissues, resulting in weakened support for the pelvic organs.

Chronic coughing can also cause other problems that can exacerbate pelvic floor dysfunction. For example, coughing can lead to increased intra-abdominal pressure, which can worsen urinary incontinence and prolapse. It can also cause irritation and inflammation of the bladder, which can lead to urgency and frequency of urination.

Treating chronic coughing is an important part of managing pelvic floor dysfunction. The first step is to identify the underlying cause of the cough and treat it appropriately. For example, if the cough is caused by allergies, antihistamines or allergy shots may be helpful. If the cough is caused by asthma or COPD, bronchodilators or other medications may be prescribed.

In addition to treating the underlying cause of the cough, there are also steps that can be taken to reduce the impact of coughing on the pelvic floor. These may include practicing pelvic floor exercises, such as Kegels, to strengthen the pelvic floor muscles. It may also be helpful to use a cough suppressant medication or to modify coughing technique to reduce the forceful contraction of the abdominal muscles.

Another important aspect of managing pelvic floor dysfunction related to chronic coughing is to practice good bladder and bowel habits. This may include scheduling regular times to empty the bladder and bowel, avoiding constipation, and maintaining a healthy diet and hydration.

In some cases, more advanced treatments may be necessary to manage pelvic floor dysfunction related to chronic coughing. These may include surgery to repair damaged pelvic floor tissues or to implant devices to support the pelvic organs. However, these treatments are typically reserved for more severe cases and are not always necessary.

Heavy lifting

Pelvic floor dysfunction is a common condition that affects millions of people worldwide. It occurs when the muscles, ligaments, and connective tissues that support the pelvic organs weaken or become damaged, leading to various symptoms. One of the common causes of pelvic floor dysfunction is heavy lifting, which puts a strain on the pelvic floor muscles and can result in a range of symptoms such as urinary incontinence, fecal incontinence, and pelvic pain.

Heavy lifting is a common activity that involves using the muscles of the body to move heavy objects. This activity can be done at work, at home, or at the gym, and can involve lifting weights, carrying heavy objects, or performing physically demanding tasks. While heavy lifting can provide a range of benefits, such as building strength and endurance, it can also put a significant strain on the pelvic floor muscles, which can lead to a range of issues.

When heavy lifting is performed, the pelvic floor muscles are put under stress. This stress can cause the muscles to weaken or become damaged, which can lead to symptoms such as urinary and fecal incontinence. In addition, heavy lifting can cause the pelvic organs to move out of their proper positions, leading to pelvic organ prolapse. This condition occurs when the pelvic organs, such as the bladder, uterus, or rectum, move out of their proper positions and into the vaginal canal. This can cause discomfort, pain, and a range of other symptoms.

One of the ways to prevent pelvic floor dysfunction caused by heavy lifting is to maintain proper form when lifting heavy objects. This means bending at the knees and using the legs to lift the object, rather than using the back or other muscles. It is also important to avoid lifting objects that are too heavy, or lifting objects for prolonged periods of time. In addition, pelvic floor exercises can help to strengthen the pelvic floor muscles and reduce the risk of pelvic floor dysfunction.

If you experience symptoms of pelvic floor dysfunction, such as urinary or fecal incontinence, pelvic pain, or pelvic organ prolapse, it is important to seek medical attention. Your healthcare provider can perform a pelvic exam to evaluate the condition of your pelvic floor muscles and determine the best course of treatment. Treatment options may include pelvic floor exercises, lifestyle modifications, and in some cases, surgery.

High-impact exercises

High-impact exercises have numerous health benefits, including improved cardiovascular health, increased strength, and weight loss. However, they can also put significant strain on the body, particularly the pelvic floor muscles. The pelvic floor is a group of muscles that support the pelvic organs, including the bladder, uterus, and rectum. When these muscles become weakened or damaged, it can lead to pelvic floor dysfunction (PFD). Below we will explore the relationship between high-impact exercises and PFD, and how to prevent and manage this condition.

High-impact exercises, such as running, jumping, and plyometrics, create a great deal of force on the pelvic floor muscles. This force can cause the muscles to become overstretched and weakened over time, leading to PFD. Symptoms of PFD include urinary incontinence, fecal incontinence, pelvic pain, and discomfort during sexual activity. Women who have given birth, are menopausal, or are overweight are particularly susceptible to PFD, and high-impact exercises can exacerbate these issues.

However, this doesn't mean that you need to give up high-impact exercises entirely. In fact, regular exercise can actually help to improve pelvic floor strength and reduce the risk of PFD. The key is to approach high-impact exercises with caution and to take steps to protect your pelvic floor.

One way to protect the pelvic floor during high-impact exercises is to engage in regular pelvic floor muscle training, also known as Kegels. Kegels involve contracting and relaxing the pelvic floor muscles, and can be done anywhere at any time. Strengthening these muscles can help to improve bladder and bowel control, reduce pelvic pain, and increase sexual satisfaction. Incorporating Kegels into your regular exercise routine can help to counteract the strain that high-impact exercises put on the pelvic floor muscles.

Another way to protect the pelvic floor during high-impact exercises is to modify your workout routine. For example, instead of running on a hard surface, try running on a softer surface such as grass or a treadmill with cushioning. This can help to reduce the impact on the pelvic floor muscles. Similarly, incorporating low-impact exercises such as swimming, cycling, or yoga into your routine can help to give the pelvic floor muscles a break from the strain of high-impact exercises.

Proper form is also important when it comes to protecting the pelvic floor during high-impact exercises. For example, when doing jumping jacks or other jumping exercises, make sure to land softly on your feet and to engage your pelvic floor muscles as you land. This can help to reduce the impact on the pelvic floor muscles and prevent damage.

It is also important to listen to your body when it comes to high-impact exercises. If you are experiencing pelvic pain or discomfort during a workout, take a break and consult with a healthcare provider. They may recommend modifications to your workout routine or other interventions to help manage PFD.

Genetics

Pelvic floor dysfunction (PFD) is a common condition that affects both men and women, but it is more prevalent in women. It refers to a range of problems that arise from weakened, stretched, or damaged pelvic floor muscles. These muscles are crucial in supporting the bladder, uterus, and rectum, and if they become compromised, they can lead to a range of symptoms, including urinary incontinence, fecal incontinence, and pelvic pain. While the causes of pelvic floor dysfunction can be varied and complex, research has shown that genetics may play a role in predisposing some individuals to the condition.

To understand the relationship between genetics and PFD, it is first essential to understand the anatomy of the pelvic floor. The pelvic floor is made up of layers of muscles and connective tissue that stretch like a hammock from the pubic bone to the tailbone. These muscles are responsible for supporting the pelvic organs and controlling the openings of the urethra, vagina, and anus. Any weakness or damage to these muscles can result in PFD.

Research has shown that there may be a genetic component to PFD. A study published in the Journal of Urology found that a specific gene variant, COL3A1, is associated with pelvic organ prolapse, which is a form of PFD. This gene codes for type III collagen, a protein that plays a crucial role in the strength and elasticity of connective tissue throughout the body, including in the pelvic floor. Mutations in the COL3A1 gene can lead to weakened connective tissue, which may increase the risk of developing pelvic organ prolapse.

In addition to genetic mutations, variations in gene expression may also play a role in the development of PFD. A study published in the American Journal of Obstetrics and Gynecology found that women with pelvic organ prolapse had lower levels of gene expression for specific collagen types compared to women without the condition. This suggests that alterations in gene expression may contribute to weakened connective tissue in the pelvic floor and increase the risk of PFD.

While genetics may predispose some individuals to PFD, environmental factors and lifestyle choices can also play a significant role in the development of the condition. For example, chronic constipation, chronic coughing, and high-impact exercise can all place excessive strain on the pelvic floor muscles, leading to weakening and damage over time. These factors can be exacerbated by genetic predispositions and lead to an increased risk of developing PFD.

Chapter Four

Diagnosis of Pelvic Floor Disorders

Pelvic floor disorders are a common problem affecting many individuals, particularly women. These disorders can result from a variety of causes, including childbirth, aging, and obesity, and can cause a range of symptoms, including urinary and fecal incontinence, constipation, and pelvic pain. Effective management of pelvic floor disorders requires an accurate diagnosis, which can be challenging due to the complex nature of these conditions. Below we will discuss the various methods used to diagnose pelvic floor disorders.

One of the most commonly used diagnostic methods for pelvic floor disorders is a physical examination. This examination is usually performed by a healthcare professional who specializes in treating pelvic floor disorders, such as a urogynecologist or a urologist. During the examination, the healthcare professional will assess the strength and coordination of the pelvic floor muscles, as well as the integrity of the pelvic organs. They will also evaluate the patient's ability to contract and relax their pelvic floor muscles, which can help determine the presence and severity of any pelvic floor dysfunction.

Another commonly used diagnostic method for pelvic floor disorders is imaging studies, such as magnetic resonance imaging (MRI) and ultrasound. These imaging studies can help identify structural abnormalities in the pelvic region, such as prolapse of pelvic organs, which can contribute to pelvic floor dysfunction. MRI and ultrasound can also provide information about the strength and integrity of the pelvic floor muscles, which can help guide treatment decisions.

In some cases, specialized tests may be needed to diagnose pelvic floor disorders. One such test is urodynamics, which is a series of tests used to evaluate the function of the urinary system. During urodynamics, a small tube is inserted into the bladder to measure the pressure inside. The patient is then asked to cough or perform other activities to assess the coordination between the bladder and pelvic floor muscles. Urodynamics can help identify the presence of urinary incontinence and provide information about the severity of the problem.

Another specialized test used to diagnose pelvic floor disorders is defecography. This test involves the use of a special x-ray to visualize the rectum and anus as the patient attempts to defecate. Defecography can provide information about the presence of pelvic organ prolapse and the coordination between the pelvic floor muscles and the rectum.

In addition to these diagnostic methods, healthcare professionals may also use questionnaires or surveys to assess the patient's symptoms and quality of life. These questionnaires can provide valuable information about the impact of pelvic floor disorders on daily life and can help guide treatment decisions.

In some cases, healthcare professionals may also use a combination of these diagnostic methods to accurately diagnose pelvic floor disorders. For example, a patient may undergo a physical examination and imaging studies to identify the presence of pelvic organ prolapse, followed by urodynamics to evaluate the function of the urinary system.

Pelvic exam

Pelvic exams are an important part of a woman's healthcare routine. During a pelvic exam, a healthcare provider examines the pelvic organs, including the uterus, cervix, ovaries, fallopian tubes, bladder, and rectum. Pelvic exams are crucial in the diagnosis of pelvic floor disorders, including pelvic floor dysfunction.

Pelvic floor dysfunction is a common condition that affects many women. The pelvic floor is a group of muscles and ligaments that support the pelvic organs. When the pelvic floor muscles become weakened or damaged, it can result in a range of symptoms, including urinary incontinence, fecal incontinence, pelvic pain, and discomfort during sexual intercourse. Pelvic floor dysfunction can be caused by a range of factors, including pregnancy and childbirth, aging, obesity, and chronic coughing.

Pelvic exams can help healthcare providers diagnose pelvic floor disorders. During a pelvic exam, a healthcare provider can assess the strength and tone of the pelvic floor muscles. They can also evaluate the position and size of the pelvic organs, as well as check for any signs of inflammation, infection, or abnormalities.

The first step in a pelvic exam is to review the patient's medical history. The healthcare provider will ask questions about the patient's symptoms, medical history, and any medications they are taking. They may also ask about their sexual history and whether they have had any surgeries or medical procedures that may affect the pelvic organs.

After reviewing the patient's medical history, the healthcare provider will perform a physical exam. They will begin by examining the external genitalia, including the labia and clitoris. Next, they will insert a speculum into the vagina to view the cervix. The healthcare provider will then use their fingers to feel for any abnormalities in the vaginal walls or the pelvic organs.

During the pelvic exam, the healthcare provider may also perform a rectal exam. This involves inserting a gloved finger into the rectum to check for any abnormalities in the rectal walls or the pelvic floor muscles.

In some cases, a healthcare provider may also perform imaging tests to diagnose pelvic floor disorders. This may include an ultrasound, MRI, or CT scan. These tests can provide detailed images of the pelvic organs and help healthcare providers identify any abnormalities or damage to the pelvic floor muscles.

Pelvic exams can be uncomfortable or even painful for some women, but they are an important part of maintaining good pelvic health. It is important for women to schedule regular pelvic exams as part of their healthcare routine, particularly if they are experiencing symptoms of pelvic floor dysfunction.

In addition to pelvic exams, there are a range of other diagnostic tests that can be used to diagnose pelvic floor disorders. These may include urodynamic testing, which measures the function of the bladder and urethra, and cystoscopy, which involves using a thin, flexible tube with a camera to view the inside of the bladder.

Ultrasound

Ultrasound is a commonly used diagnostic tool for various medical conditions. In the context of pelvic floor dysfunction, it can be used to assess the structures and function of the pelvic floor muscles, bladder, and other pelvic organs. Below we will explore the use of ultrasound in the diagnosis of pelvic floor disorders, its benefits, and limitations.

The pelvic floor is a complex structure of muscles, ligaments, and connective tissues that supports the pelvic organs, including the bladder, uterus, and rectum. Dysfunction of these muscles can lead to a range of problems, including urinary and fecal incontinence, pelvic organ prolapse, and sexual dysfunction. Pelvic floor dysfunction affects a significant number of women worldwide, and diagnosis of this condition is essential to manage the symptoms effectively.

Ultrasound is a non-invasive imaging technique that uses high-frequency sound waves to create images of the internal organs. In pelvic floor disorders, ultrasound can be used to assess the pelvic organs' anatomy and function, as well as the pelvic floor muscles' structure and mobility. There are two main types of ultrasound used in pelvic floor imaging: transabdominal and transperineal.

Transabdominal ultrasound involves placing a probe on the abdomen to visualize the pelvic organs. This method is commonly used in the early stages of pregnancy to confirm the pregnancy's location and monitor fetal development. However, it is less useful for assessing pelvic floor muscle function and structure.

Transperineal ultrasound, on the other hand, involves inserting a small probe into the vagina or rectum to visualize the pelvic floor muscles and other pelvic organs. This method provides a more detailed view of the pelvic floor muscles' structure and function, making it a useful tool for diagnosing pelvic floor dysfunction.

The benefits of using ultrasound in the diagnosis of pelvic floor disorders are numerous. Ultrasound is a safe, non-invasive, and painless procedure that does not require exposure to radiation. It is readily available in most medical facilities and can be performed quickly and easily. Furthermore, ultrasound is a cost-effective alternative to more invasive diagnostic procedures, such as magnetic resonance imaging (MRI) or computed tomography (CT) scans.

In addition to diagnosing pelvic floor disorders, ultrasound can also be used to monitor the effectiveness of pelvic floor muscle training (PFMT). PFMT is a type of physical therapy that involves exercises designed to strengthen the pelvic floor muscles. Ultrasound can be used to visualize the pelvic floor muscles during PFMT and assess the progress of the therapy.

Despite its benefits, ultrasound has some limitations when used in the diagnosis of pelvic floor disorders. For example, the quality of the images obtained can be affected by factors such as obesity or the presence of gas in the intestines. In some cases, additional imaging techniques, such as MRI or CT scans, may be required to obtain a more accurate diagnosis.

Another limitation of ultrasound is the need for specialized training to interpret the images correctly. A skilled and experienced operator is required to obtain high-quality images and interpret them accurately. Furthermore, the interpretation of ultrasound images can be subjective, and different operators may interpret the images differently.

X-rays

X-rays are a commonly used imaging technique that can be helpful in diagnosing a variety of medical conditions, including pelvic floor dysfunction. The pelvic floor is a group of muscles, ligaments, and tissues that support the organs in the pelvis, including the bladder, uterus, and rectum. When these muscles become weak or damaged, it can lead to a range of symptoms, such as incontinence, pelvic pain, and sexual dysfunction. X-rays can help doctors visualize the structures of the pelvis and identify any issues that may be causing pelvic floor dysfunction.

X-rays work by using electromagnetic radiation to create images of the body. During the procedure, the patient will lie on a table while a specialized x-ray machine is positioned over the pelvic area. The machine emits a small amount of radiation, which passes through the body and is absorbed differently by the various tissues in the pelvis. This creates an image on a digital or film screen, which can be viewed by the doctor.

X-rays are commonly used to diagnose pelvic floor dysfunction, as they can provide detailed images of the bones and organs in the pelvis. They can help doctors identify any abnormalities or damage to the pelvic bones, such as fractures or dislocations, that may be contributing to the patient's symptoms. X-rays can also be used to evaluate the position and size of the pelvic organs, such as the bladder and uterus, and determine if they are causing any issues with the pelvic floor.

X-rays can also be useful in diagnosing specific types of pelvic floor dysfunction, such as rectocele and cystocele. A rectocele occurs when the rectum bulges into the back of the vagina, while a cystocele occurs when the bladder bulges into the front of the vagina. X-rays can help doctors visualize the extent of the bulge and determine the severity of the condition.

One type of x-ray that is commonly used to diagnose pelvic floor dysfunction is called a voiding cystourethrogram (VCUG). During this procedure, a catheter is inserted into the bladder through the urethra, and a contrast dye is injected into the bladder. The patient will then be asked to urinate, while x-rays are taken to visualize the flow of urine and identify any issues with the urinary tract.

While x-rays can be helpful in diagnosing pelvic floor dysfunction, there are some risks associated with the procedure. X-rays use a small amount of radiation, which can potentially increase the risk of cancer over time. However, the amount of radiation used in diagnostic x-rays is generally considered safe, and the benefits of the procedure usually outweigh the risks.

In addition, x-rays may not always provide a complete picture of the pelvic floor. They are not able to visualize soft tissues, such as muscles and ligaments, as well as other imaging techniques, such as magnetic resonance imaging (MRI) or ultrasound. These imaging techniques may be used in combination with x-rays to provide a more comprehensive diagnosis.

MRI

Magnetic Resonance Imaging (MRI) is a non-invasive diagnostic tool used to produce detailed images of the internal structures of the body. MRI uses a powerful magnet, radio waves, and a computer to create high-resolution images of the soft tissues, bones, and organs. In recent years, MRI has become an important tool in the diagnosis and treatment of pelvic floor disorders, including pelvic organ prolapse, urinary incontinence, and fecal incontinence.

MRI is particularly useful in diagnosing pelvic floor disorders because it can provide highly detailed images of the pelvic area, allowing doctors to see the pelvic organs and muscles in great detail. MRI can help doctors to identify the extent of pelvic organ prolapse, determine the cause of urinary or fecal incontinence, and identify other issues such as tumors or abnormal growths that may be affecting the pelvic organs.

There are several different types of MRI scans that can be used to diagnose pelvic floor disorders. The most common type of MRI used for pelvic imaging is a T2-weighted image, which provides a high level of detail of the soft tissues in the pelvis. This type of scan can show the location and size of pelvic organs, such as the bladder, uterus, and rectum, as well as the pelvic floor muscles and ligaments.

Another type of MRI that can be used to diagnose pelvic floor disorders is a dynamic MRI, also known as a cine MRI. This type of MRI involves taking multiple images of the pelvis while the patient is in different positions or performing specific movements, such as coughing or bearing down. These images can help doctors to see how the pelvic organs and muscles move during different activities, which can provide important information about the cause of pelvic floor dysfunction.

MRI can also be used to assess the structure and function of the pelvic floor muscles. One technique that can be used is called magnetic resonance defecography. This involves having the patient sit on a special toilet while undergoing an MRI scan. The scan can show how the pelvic organs move during defecation, which can help doctors to identify any problems with the muscles or nerves that control bowel movements.

MRI is a safe and non-invasive procedure, but there are some precautions that need to be taken. Patients with certain types of medical devices, such as pacemakers or cochlear implants, may not be able to undergo an MRI scan. Additionally, pregnant women should avoid MRI scans during the first trimester, as there is a small risk of harm to the developing fetus.

Urodynamics testing

Pelvic floor dysfunction (PFD) can be a frustrating and sometimes debilitating condition that affects millions of people worldwide. Symptoms of PFD include urinary and fecal incontinence, pelvic pain, and difficulty emptying the bladder or bowels. Diagnosing PFD can be a challenge, but urodynamic testing is a valuable tool in identifying the specific type of dysfunction present and developing a treatment plan.

Urodynamic testing is a type of diagnostic testing used to evaluate how well the bladder and urethra are functioning. It is often used to diagnose and evaluate conditions such as urinary incontinence, urinary tract infections, and bladder dysfunction. The test is performed in a hospital or clinic setting and is typically done on an outpatient basis. Urodynamic testing is usually done by a urologist or urogynecologist, who is a specialist in treating disorders of the urinary tract and pelvic floor.

The urodynamic testing procedure involves several different tests that are designed to evaluate how well the bladder and urethra are functioning. These tests may include uroflowmetry, cystometry, and pressure flow studies.

Uroflowmetry measures the rate and amount of urine flow during voiding. A person will be asked to urinate into a special device that measures the speed and volume of the urine flow. This test can help identify problems with urine flow, such as obstruction or weakness in the pelvic floor muscles.

Cystometry measures the pressure inside the bladder as it fills and empties. A catheter is inserted into the bladder, and a sterile fluid is infused to fill the bladder. The pressure in the bladder is then measured as the person urinates or is asked to cough or bear down. This test can help diagnose bladder dysfunction, such as overactive bladder or underactive bladder.

Pressure flow studies are a more detailed version of cystometry. This test measures the pressure inside the bladder and the flow rate of urine during voiding. It can help diagnose the specific type of urinary incontinence a person may be experiencing, such as stress incontinence or urge incontinence.

Urodynamic testing can be uncomfortable, but it is usually not painful. The test may take up to an hour or more to complete, depending on the specific tests being done. The urologist or urogynecologist will review the results of the tests and develop a treatment plan based on the specific type of dysfunction present.

The most common treatments for PFD include pelvic floor exercises, medications, and surgery. Pelvic floor exercises, also known as Kegels, involve contracting and relaxing the muscles that control the bladder and bowel. These exercises can strengthen the pelvic floor muscles and improve bladder and bowel control. Medications may be used to treat overactive bladder or other types of urinary incontinence. Surgery may be an option for more severe cases of PFD, such as those caused by a prolapsed bladder or rectum.

Chapter Five

Treatment Options for Pelvic Floor Disorders

Pelvic floor dysfunction (PFD) is a common condition among women that affects the muscles, ligaments, and connective tissues of the pelvic floor. The pelvic floor muscles provide support to the bladder, uterus, and rectum. These muscles may weaken over time due to various factors like childbirth, aging, chronic constipation, obesity, and heavy lifting. PFD can cause a range of symptoms like urinary or fecal incontinence, difficulty with bowel movements, pelvic pain, and sexual dysfunction. Treatment options for PFD vary depending on the severity of symptoms and underlying causes. Below we will explore various treatment options available for PFD.

Pelvic floor exercises

Pelvic floor exercises are also known as Kegel exercises. These exercises involve repeatedly contracting and relaxing the pelvic floor muscles to strengthen them. These exercises can help improve bladder and bowel control, reduce pelvic pain, and improve sexual function. Pelvic floor exercises are often the first line of treatment for mild to moderate PFD. A physical therapist specialized in pelvic floor rehabilitation can guide women on how to perform these exercises correctly.

Biofeedback

Biofeedback is a technique used to monitor the muscle activity of the pelvic floor during Kegel exercises. A biofeedback machine measures the strength and duration of muscle contractions and provides visual or auditory feedback to help women perform these exercises more effectively. Biofeedback can help women learn how to contract and relax their pelvic floor muscles correctly.

Electrical stimulation

Electrical stimulation is a technique used to improve muscle strength in the pelvic floor. An electrode is placed in the vagina or anus, and a mild electrical current is used to stimulate the muscles. Electrical stimulation can help improve muscle strength and reduce symptoms of urinary or fecal incontinence.

Medications

Medications can be used to treat certain symptoms of PFD. For example, anticholinergic medications can help reduce urinary urgency and frequency. Muscle relaxants can be used to reduce pelvic pain and discomfort.

Surgery

Surgery may be an option for severe cases of PFD, where other treatments have failed. Surgery can involve repairing damaged tissues, strengthening weak muscles, or removing excess tissue. There are several surgical procedures available for PFD, including slings, mesh implants, and colposuspension.

Behavioral modifications

Behavioral modifications can help reduce symptoms of PFD. These modifications include dietary changes, such as increasing fiber intake, reducing caffeine and alcohol consumption, and avoiding constipation. Weight loss can also help reduce symptoms of PFD in overweight women. Women with PFD should avoid activities that can strain the pelvic floor, like heavy lifting, high-impact exercises, and long periods of sitting.

Pelvic floor physical therapy

Pelvic floor physical therapy involves working with a physical therapist specialized in pelvic floor rehabilitation. The therapist can provide exercises, manual therapy, and behavioral modifications tailored to the individual's needs. Pelvic floor physical therapy can help reduce symptoms of PFD, improve muscle strength and flexibility, and improve quality of life.

Pelvic floor exercises (Kegels)

Pelvic floor muscles play a vital role in supporting the organs in the pelvis, such as the bladder, uterus, and rectum. Pelvic floor dysfunction is a common condition that affects many individuals, particularly women. Symptoms of pelvic floor dysfunction may include urinary and fecal incontinence, pelvic pain, and sexual dysfunction. Pelvic floor exercises, also known as Kegel exercises, are one of the most effective treatment options for pelvic floor disorders.

Kegel exercises are named after Dr. Arnold Kegel, who first introduced the exercise in the late 1940s to help women who experienced incontinence after childbirth. Kegel exercises involve repeatedly contracting and relaxing the muscles that form the pelvic floor. These exercises help to strengthen the pelvic floor muscles, which can improve bladder and bowel control, reduce pelvic pain, and enhance sexual function.

To perform Kegel exercises, individuals need to identify the pelvic floor muscles first. These are the muscles that help control the urine flow and hold up the pelvic organs. To locate the pelvic floor muscles, individuals should imagine that they are trying to stop the flow of urine midstream. The muscles that are squeezed to do so are the pelvic floor muscles.

Once the pelvic floor muscles are identified, the next step is to perform the Kegel exercises. To do this, individuals should follow these steps:

Tighten the pelvic floor muscles and hold for 5 seconds.

Relax the muscles for 5 seconds.

Repeat the tightening and relaxing for 10-15 repetitions.

It is recommended to perform Kegel exercises three times a day. Gradually, individuals can work their way up to holding the contractions for 10 seconds each time.

Kegel exercises are beneficial for a variety of pelvic floor disorders. They can improve bladder and bowel control, reduce the risk of urine leakage, and prevent pelvic organ prolapse. Kegel exercises are also an effective treatment option for pelvic pain and sexual dysfunction. Research has shown that regular Kegel exercises can improve the strength and endurance of the pelvic floor muscles, leading to improved overall pelvic health.

In addition to Kegel exercises, there are other treatments available for pelvic floor disorders. For instance, biofeedback therapy, in which an individual receives feedback about the strength and coordination of their pelvic floor muscles, can help individuals learn how to properly perform Kegel exercises. Other treatments may include medication, dietary changes, and surgery.

It is important to note that Kegel exercises may not be appropriate for everyone. Individuals who have difficulty identifying their pelvic floor muscles or who have a weakened pelvic floor may need to work with a physical therapist to properly perform the exercises. Additionally, overexertion of the pelvic floor muscles can also lead to pelvic pain or muscle spasm. Therefore, it is important to consult a healthcare provider before starting a new exercise program.

Biofeedback

Biofeedback is a non-invasive therapy that is becoming increasingly popular in the management of pelvic floor dysfunction. Pelvic floor dysfunction is a broad term used to describe a range of conditions that affect the pelvic floor muscles. The pelvic floor muscles are responsible for supporting the organs within the pelvis and for controlling the bladder, bowel, and sexual functions. When these muscles become weak or dysfunctional, it can lead to a range of symptoms, including urinary and fecal incontinence, pelvic pain, and sexual dysfunction.

Biofeedback is a technique used to improve the function of the pelvic floor muscles. It involves using sensors to monitor the activity of the muscles and providing feedback to the patient. The feedback can be visual, auditory, or tactile and is designed to help the patient understand how to correctly contract and relax their pelvic floor muscles. Biofeedback is often used in combination with other therapies, such as pelvic floor exercises (Kegels) and electrical stimulation, to improve the overall effectiveness of treatment.

Biofeedback can be performed in a clinical setting or at home with a portable device. In a clinical setting, the patient is connected to a machine that measures the activity of the pelvic floor muscles. The machine displays the activity of the muscles on a screen, allowing the patient to see how their muscles are contracting and relaxing. The patient is then instructed on how to contract and relax their muscles correctly, and the machine provides feedback on the effectiveness of the contractions.

In the home setting, the patient is provided with a small device that measures the activity of the pelvic floor muscles. The device is placed inside the vagina or rectum and is connected to a mobile app or computer. The app or computer displays the activity of the muscles and provides feedback to the patient. The patient can use the device at home to perform pelvic floor exercises and monitor their progress over time.

Biofeedback has been shown to be an effective therapy for the management of pelvic floor dysfunction. Studies have shown that biofeedback can improve the strength and endurance of the pelvic floor muscles, reduce symptoms of urinary and fecal incontinence, and improve sexual function.

Biofeedback is a safe and non-invasive therapy that can be used in combination with other treatments for pelvic floor dysfunction. It is important to note that biofeedback may not be suitable for all patients, and a thorough evaluation by a healthcare professional is necessary before starting any treatment.

One of the benefits of biofeedback is that it is a personalized therapy. The feedback provided to the patient is tailored to their specific needs and allows them to focus on improving their individual weaknesses. This personalized approach can lead to better outcomes and improved patient satisfaction.

In addition to improving the function of the pelvic floor muscles, biofeedback can also be used to address other conditions that affect the muscles of the body, such as chronic pain and muscle tension. Biofeedback can help patients learn to control their muscle tension and reduce the symptoms associated with these conditions.

Electrical stimulation

Electrical stimulation, also known as neuromuscular electrical stimulation (NMES), is a non-invasive treatment option for pelvic floor dysfunction. Pelvic floor dysfunction can be caused by a variety of factors such as childbirth, aging, obesity, and nerve damage. It can lead to symptoms such as urinary incontinence, fecal incontinence, and pelvic pain. Electrical stimulation is one of the many treatments available for pelvic floor dysfunction and it works by sending small electrical impulses to the pelvic floor muscles to improve their strength and function.

Electrical stimulation can be performed in different ways. One method involves the use of a small device that is inserted into the vagina or rectum. The device is connected to electrodes that are placed on the skin near the pelvic floor muscles. Another method involves the use of external electrodes that are placed on the skin near the pelvic floor muscles.

The electrical impulses generated by the device cause the pelvic floor muscles to contract and relax in a pattern that is similar to natural muscle contractions. This helps to strengthen the muscles and improve their function. Electrical stimulation can also increase blood flow to the pelvic region, which can help to promote healing and reduce inflammation.

Electrical stimulation can be used to treat a variety of pelvic floor disorders, including urinary incontinence, fecal incontinence, and pelvic pain. It can be used alone or in combination with other treatments, such as pelvic floor exercises (Kegels) and biofeedback.

Studies have shown that electrical stimulation can be an effective treatment for urinary incontinence. In one study, women with stress urinary incontinence were treated with either electrical stimulation or pelvic floor exercises. Both groups showed significant improvement, but the women who received electrical stimulation had a greater reduction in urinary leakage.

Electrical stimulation has also been shown to be effective in the treatment of fecal incontinence. In one study, patients with fecal incontinence were treated with either electrical stimulation or biofeedback. Both groups showed significant improvement, but the patients who received electrical stimulation had a greater reduction in episodes of fecal incontinence.

In addition to its effectiveness in treating pelvic floor dysfunction, electrical stimulation is also a safe and non-invasive treatment option. It has few side effects and can be performed in a clinical setting or at home with the guidance of a healthcare provider.

However, electrical stimulation is not suitable for everyone. It should not be used in patients with pacemakers or other implanted devices, as the electrical impulses can interfere with their function. It should also not be used in patients with certain medical conditions, such as epilepsy or cancer.

Medications

Medications are one of the treatment options available for managing pelvic floor dysfunction. Below we will explore the medications used to treat pelvic floor disorders.

Anticholinergics are medications that block the action of acetylcholine, a neurotransmitter that stimulates smooth muscle contraction. They are commonly used to treat overactive bladder, which is a common symptom of pelvic floor dysfunction. Anticholinergics work by relaxing the bladder muscle, reducing the frequency of urination, and increasing bladder capacity. They are effective in reducing urinary urgency and incontinence but may cause side effects such as dry mouth, constipation, and blurred vision. Examples of anticholinergics used for the treatment of overactive bladder include oxybutynin, tolterodine, and solifenacin.

Alpha-blockers are medications that relax smooth muscle in the bladder neck and prostate, improving urine flow and reducing symptoms of urinary obstruction. They are commonly used to treat benign prostatic hyperplasia, a condition that can contribute to pelvic floor dysfunction in men. Alpha-blockers can also be used to treat women with pelvic floor dysfunction, especially those with urinary retention. The most commonly used alpha-blocker for the treatment of pelvic floor dysfunction is tamsulosin.

Tricyclic antidepressants are medications commonly used to treat depression, anxiety, and chronic pain. They are also used in the treatment of pelvic floor dysfunction. Tricyclic antidepressants work by increasing the levels of certain neurotransmitters, such as serotonin and norepinephrine, which can help to alleviate pelvic pain and improve bladder control. They can also be used to treat urinary urgency and frequency. Tricyclic antidepressants can cause side effects such as dry mouth, constipation, and drowsiness. Examples of tricyclic antidepressants used in the treatment of pelvic floor dysfunction include amitriptyline and nortriptyline.

Selective serotonin reuptake inhibitors (SSRIs) are another class of antidepressants that can be used in the treatment of pelvic floor dysfunction. They work by increasing the levels of serotonin in the brain, which can help to alleviate pain and improve mood. SSRIs can also be used to treat urinary urgency and frequency. Common side effects of SSRIs include nausea, diarrhea, and sexual dysfunction. Examples of SSRIs used in the treatment of pelvic floor dysfunction include fluoxetine and sertraline.

Estrogen therapy is a treatment option for women with pelvic floor dysfunction caused by menopause. Estrogen is a hormone that helps to maintain the health of the urogenital tract. After menopause, the levels of estrogen in the body decrease, which can lead to thinning and drying of the vaginal tissues, urinary incontinence, and urinary tract infections. Estrogen therapy can help to relieve these symptoms by restoring the levels of estrogen in the body. Estrogen can be administered in the form of vaginal creams, tablets, or rings.

Botox injections are a relatively new treatment option for overactive bladder caused by pelvic floor dysfunction. Botox is a toxin that works by blocking the release of acetylcholine, a neurotransmitter that stimulates muscle contraction. By injecting Botox into the bladder muscle, the muscle is relaxed, reducing the frequency of urination and increasing bladder capacity. Botox injections can provide long-lasting relief from overactive bladder symptoms, but they can cause side effects such as urinary retention and urinary tract infections. Patients may need to use a catheter temporarily if they experience difficulty emptying their bladder after the procedure.

The medications used to treat pelvic floor dysfunction aim to alleviate symptoms such as urinary incontinence, overactive bladder, pelvic pain, and urinary retention. The choice of medication depends on the specific symptoms and conditions being treated, as well as the patient's overall health and preference. It's important for patients to work closely with their healthcare provider to determine the most appropriate medication for their situation, taking into account the potential benefits and side effects.

Patients should also be aware that medication is often most effective when combined with other treatment options, such as pelvic floor exercises, physical therapy, and lifestyle modifications. By adopting a comprehensive treatment approach, individuals with pelvic floor dysfunction can achieve better symptom management and improve their quality of life.

Surgery

Pelvic floor dysfunction can cause discomfort, embarrassment, and even serious health issues for both men and women. While non-invasive treatments like pelvic floor exercises, biofeedback, and medications can be effective, some patients may require surgery to resolve their symptoms. Below we will we'll take a closer look at surgical options for pelvic floor dysfunction.

Pelvic floor disorders can occur due to a variety of reasons, including childbirth, aging, hormonal changes, and injury. These disorders can affect both men and women and can lead to symptoms such as urinary or fecal incontinence, chronic constipation, pelvic pain, and sexual dysfunction.

When non-invasive treatments such as pelvic floor exercises and medications do not provide relief, surgery may be necessary. Surgery for pelvic floor disorders typically involves repairing or strengthening the pelvic floor muscles or the tissues that support them.

One common type of surgery for pelvic floor dysfunction is a sling procedure. This procedure involves placing a sling, or a strip of synthetic mesh or tissue, under the urethra or bladder neck to provide support and prevent stress urinary incontinence. The sling can be placed through a small incision in the vaginal wall or through the abdomen.

Another type of surgery for pelvic floor dysfunction is a colposuspension. This procedure involves lifting and repositioning the bladder neck to improve support and prevent stress urinary incontinence. This can be done through an incision in the abdomen or laparoscopically, using a small camera and instruments inserted through small incisions in the abdomen.

For women with pelvic organ prolapse, which occurs when the muscles and tissues supporting the pelvic organs weaken and the organs descend into the vaginal canal, there are several surgical options. One option is a hysterectomy, which involves removing the uterus to alleviate pressure on the pelvic floor muscles. Another option is a sacrocolpopexy, which involves using a piece of mesh to support the pelvic organs and lift them back into their normal position. This procedure can be done through an incision in the abdomen or laparoscopically.

In addition to these procedures, there are other surgical options for pelvic floor dysfunction, such as sphincteroplasty for anal incontinence and perineal repair for perineal tears or injuries. Each patient's treatment plan will be tailored to their individual needs and may involve a combination of non-invasive and surgical treatments.

While surgery can be effective for treating pelvic floor dysfunction, it does carry some risks. These risks include infection, bleeding, and damage to nearby organs. Patients should discuss the risks and benefits of surgery with their healthcare provider before making a decision.

It's also important to note that surgery is not always a permanent solution for pelvic floor dysfunction. While it can provide relief for many patients, the underlying condition may still be present and may require ongoing treatment.

Chapter Six

Exercises to Strengthen the Pelvic Floor

The pelvic floor muscles are essential for maintaining good bladder, bowel, and sexual function. However, many women experience pelvic floor dysfunction due to childbirth, menopause, and other factors. Fortunately, there are several exercises that can be done to strengthen the pelvic floor muscles and alleviate symptoms. Below we will discuss some of the best exercises to strengthen the pelvic floor muscles.

Kegels

Kegel exercises are one of the most popular pelvic floor exercises. They are named after Dr. Arnold Kegel, who first described the exercises in the 1940s. Kegels involve contracting and relaxing the pelvic floor muscles. To do Kegels, sit comfortably and squeeze the muscles as if you were trying to stop the flow of urine. Hold for a few seconds, then release. Repeat this process 10-15 times per session, and aim to do 3-4 sessions per day.

Squats

Squats are a great exercise for strengthening the pelvic floor muscles as they work the glutes and hips. Stand with your feet shoulder-width apart, and lower yourself down into a squatting position. Be sure to keep your knees behind your toes, and your weight on your heels. Hold this position for a few seconds, then rise back up to the starting position. Repeat this exercise 10-15 times per session, and aim to do 3-4 sessions per day.

Lunges

Lunges are another great exercise for strengthening the pelvic floor muscles. Stand with your feet shoulder-width apart and take a big step forward with one foot. Lower your body down until your front knee is at a 90-degree angle, then rise back up to the starting position. Repeat this process with the other leg. Aim to do 10-15 reps per leg per session, and aim to do 3-4 sessions per day.

Bridges

Bridges work the glutes and hips, which are important for maintaining good pelvic floor muscle strength. Lie on your back with your knees bent and your feet flat on the floor. Raise your hips up towards the ceiling, making sure to engage your glutes and pelvic floor muscles. Hold this position for a few seconds, then lower back down to the starting position. Repeat this exercise 10-15 times per session, and aim to do 3-4 sessions per day.

Pelvic tilts

Pelvic tilts are a simple but effective exercise for strengthening the pelvic floor muscles. Lie on your back with your knees bent and your feet flat on the floor. Slowly tilt your pelvis up towards the ceiling, then back down to the floor. Repeat this exercise 10-15 times per session, and aim to do 3-4 sessions per day.

Deadlifts

Deadlifts work the glutes, hips, and lower back, making them a great exercise for strengthening the pelvic floor muscles. Stand with your feet shoulder-width apart and a weight in your hands. Bend down at the hips and lower the weight towards the floor, making sure to keep your back straight and your weight on your heels. Rise back up to the starting position, squeezing your glutes and pelvic floor muscles as you do so. Repeat this exercise 10-15 times per session, and aim to do 3-4 sessions per day.

Kegel exercises

One of the most effective ways to treat PFD is through pelvic floor muscle exercises, also known as Kegel exercises. Below we will explore what Kegel exercises are, how they work, and how they can benefit individuals with pelvic floor dysfunction.

Kegel exercises are named after Arnold Kegel, an American gynecologist who first described them in the 1940s. The exercises involve contracting and relaxing the muscles of the pelvic floor, which support the bladder, uterus, and rectum. These muscles can weaken over time due to factors such as aging, pregnancy, childbirth, obesity, and certain medical conditions. Weakening of the pelvic floor muscles can lead to PFD symptoms such as urinary and fecal incontinence, pelvic organ prolapse, and sexual dysfunction.

Kegel exercises work by strengthening the pelvic floor muscles, which can help to improve bladder and bowel control, reduce pelvic pain, and enhance sexual function. The exercises can be performed by both men and women and are simple to do. To perform a Kegel exercise, individuals should first identify their pelvic floor muscles. This can be done by stopping the flow of urine midstream or by inserting a finger into the vagina or anus and contracting the muscles around it. Once the muscles are identified, individuals should contract them for 5-10 seconds, then relax for the same amount of time. The exercise can be repeated 10-15 times in a row, several times a day.

While Kegel exercises can be done anywhere, it is important to perform them correctly to achieve maximum benefit. One common mistake is using the wrong muscles or tensing other muscles, such as the buttocks or abdomen, instead of the pelvic floor muscles. Another mistake is holding the breath or straining while contracting the muscles, which can cause more harm than good. To ensure that Kegel exercises are being performed correctly, it may be helpful to consult with a healthcare provider, pelvic floor physical therapist, or certified pelvic health coach.

Kegel exercises have been shown to be effective in treating a variety of pelvic floor disorders. For example, they can help to improve urinary incontinence by strengthening the muscles that control the bladder. In one study, women who performed Kegel exercises for 8 weeks experienced significant improvements in urinary incontinence compared to a control group. Another study found that men who performed Kegel exercises after prostate surgery had better urinary control and improved sexual function compared to those who did not do the exercises.

In addition to improving bladder and bowel control, Kegel exercises can also help to reduce pelvic pain and discomfort. For example, individuals with chronic pelvic pain syndrome may benefit from performing Kegel exercises, as they can help to relax the pelvic floor muscles and improve blood flow to the area. Kegel exercises have also been shown to be effective in reducing pain and discomfort associated with vulvodynia, a chronic pain condition that affects the vulva.

Kegel exercises can also be beneficial for individuals experiencing sexual dysfunction, such as erectile dysfunction or painful intercourse. By strengthening the pelvic floor muscles, Kegel exercises can improve blood flow to the genital area and enhance sexual arousal and pleasure. In one study, women who performed Kegel exercises reported increased sexual desire and satisfaction compared to a control group.

While Kegel exercises are generally safe, there are some situations in which they may not be appropriate or may need to be modified. For example, individuals with certain medical conditions such as pelvic organ prolapse or a urinary tract infection may need to avoid or adjust their Kegel exercise routine. Additionally, individuals who experience pain during Kegel exercises should stop immediately and consult a healthcare provider to ensure they are performing the exercises correctly and to rule out any underlying conditions that may need to be addressed.

To maximize the benefits of Kegel exercises, consistency is key. Regular practice, ideally daily, is important for strengthening the pelvic floor muscles and achieving long-term improvements in symptoms. However, it may take several weeks or even months of consistent practice to notice significant changes, so patience and persistence are essential.

Incorporating Kegel exercises into a broader pelvic floor rehabilitation program can also enhance their effectiveness. This may include additional exercises to strengthen the core and pelvic muscles, biofeedback therapy to improve awareness and control of the pelvic floor muscles, and lifestyle changes such as dietary modifications to manage weight and prevent constipation, which can put additional strain on the pelvic floor.

Overall, Kegel exercises offer a non-invasive, effective way to treat and manage symptoms of pelvic floor dysfunction. By strengthening the pelvic floor muscles, individuals can improve their bladder and bowel control, reduce pelvic pain, and enhance their sexual function and overall quality of life. With proper technique, consistent practice, and guidance from healthcare professionals when needed, Kegel exercises can be a valuable tool in the management of pelvic floor dysfunction.

Kegel Balls

Kegel exercises are a popular way of strengthening the pelvic floor muscles to treat and prevent pelvic floor dysfunction. However, for those who find it challenging to perform Kegels correctly, there is another option: Kegel balls. Below we will discuss what Kegel balls are, how they work, and their effectiveness in treating pelvic floor dysfunction.

What are Kegel Balls?

Kegel balls, also known as Ben Wa balls, are small weighted balls that are inserted into the vagina to help women perform Kegel exercises. They are typically made of medical-grade silicone or plastic and come in a variety of sizes, shapes, and weights. The balls are connected by a string, which is used to remove them after use.

How do Kegel Balls work?

Kegel balls work by providing resistance to the pelvic floor muscles, which in turn helps to strengthen them. When the balls are inserted into the vagina, the pelvic floor muscles must contract to keep them in place. This contraction helps to strengthen the muscles over time. Additionally, the movement of the balls within the vagina can provide additional stimulation to the pelvic floor muscles, increasing their effectiveness.

Are Kegel Balls effective in treating pelvic floor dysfunction?

Studies have shown that Kegel balls can be effective in treating pelvic floor dysfunction. In a randomized controlled trial of 74 women with stress urinary incontinence, those who used Kegel balls saw a significant reduction in their symptoms compared to those who did not use them. Additionally, a study of 69 women with urinary incontinence found that Kegel balls were effective in improving pelvic floor muscle strength and reducing incontinence.

It's important to note that Kegel balls are not a one-size-fits-all solution. The weight and size of the balls used should be appropriate for the individual's level of muscle strength and comfort. Using balls that are too heavy or large can cause discomfort or even damage to the pelvic floor muscles.

How to use Kegel Balls?

Using Kegel balls is relatively simple. It's important to start with a clean and dry set of balls, and to use a water-based lubricant if needed. Begin by lying down and inserting the balls into the vagina, with the string outside the body. Contract the pelvic floor muscles to hold the balls in place for a few minutes, then release and rest for a few seconds. Repeat this process for several minutes, a few times a week. It's essential to listen to your body and stop if you experience discomfort or pain.

Squats

Squats are a popular exercise that can help strengthen the pelvic floor muscles, which can be especially beneficial for individuals with pelvic floor dysfunction. Pelvic floor dysfunction is a condition where the muscles of the pelvic floor, which support the bladder, uterus, and rectum, are weakened or damaged. This can lead to a variety of symptoms, including urinary incontinence, bowel incontinence, and pelvic pain. Fortunately, exercises like squats can help improve pelvic floor muscle strength and alleviate these symptoms.

Squats are a compound exercise, meaning they work multiple muscle groups at once. When done correctly, squats engage not only the legs and glutes but also the core and pelvic floor muscles. The movement of the squat involves lowering the body into a seated position and then standing back up again, which requires the pelvic floor muscles to contract and support the weight of the body.

To perform a squat, start by standing with feet hip-width apart and toes pointed forward. Engage the core and begin to lower the body by bending the knees and pushing the hips back as if sitting in a chair. Keep the weight in the heels and the chest lifted as the body lowers. Once the thighs are parallel to the ground, pause for a moment and then push through the heels to stand back up.

It is essential to maintain proper form when performing squats to avoid injury and maximize the benefits. One common mistake is allowing the knees to collapse inward during the movement, which can put unnecessary strain on the knees and weaken the pelvic floor muscles. Instead, focus on keeping the knees tracking over the toes and maintaining a neutral spine.

Squats can be modified to accommodate different fitness levels and pelvic floor conditions. For individuals with severe pelvic floor dysfunction or pain, it may be beneficial to start with a shallow squat and gradually work up to a full squat. It is also possible to perform squats against a wall or with a chair for added support.

Another way to modify squats is by using props like resistance bands or weights. Resistance bands can be looped around the thighs to provide extra resistance and engage the glutes and pelvic floor muscles. Similarly, holding a weight or kettlebell at chest height during the squat can increase the intensity of the exercise and target the pelvic floor muscles even more.

In addition to improving pelvic floor muscle strength, squats offer a variety of other health benefits. They can help increase bone density and prevent osteoporosis, improve balance and coordination, and burn calories and build muscle mass.

When incorporating squats into a pelvic floor exercise routine, it is important to start slowly and gradually increase the intensity and frequency of the exercise. Overtraining or pushing too hard too soon can lead to injury or exacerbate pelvic floor dysfunction symptoms.

Bridges

Bridges are a type of exercise that can help strengthen the pelvic floor muscles, which can help with pelvic floor dysfunction. Pelvic floor dysfunction refers to a variety of conditions that affect the muscles, ligaments, and tissues that support the pelvic organs, including the bladder, uterus, and rectum. These conditions can result in a variety of symptoms, including urinary incontinence, fecal incontinence, and pelvic pain. Strengthening the pelvic floor muscles can help improve these symptoms, and bridges are one exercise that can be particularly helpful in this regard.

To perform a bridge, lie on your back with your knees bent and your feet flat on the ground. Tighten your buttocks and lift your hips up towards the ceiling, keeping your feet and shoulders on the ground. Hold the position for a few seconds, then lower your hips back down to the ground. Repeat for several repetitions.

Bridges are a great exercise for strengthening the glutes, which are important muscles for supporting the pelvis. When the glutes are weak, it can put extra pressure on the pelvic floor muscles, leading to dysfunction. By strengthening the glutes, bridges can help reduce this pressure and improve pelvic floor function.

Bridges can be modified to make them easier or more difficult depending on your fitness level. For example, you can perform single-leg bridges, where you lift one foot off the ground while performing the exercise. This variation adds extra challenge to the glutes and pelvic floor muscles. Alternatively, you can use resistance bands or weights to increase the difficulty of the exercise.

While bridges are generally safe for most people, it's important to use proper form to avoid injury. Make sure to keep your feet and shoulders firmly planted on the ground and avoid arching your back. If you experience pain or discomfort while performing the exercise, stop and consult with a healthcare professional.

In addition to bridges, there are other exercises that can help strengthen the pelvic floor muscles and improve pelvic floor function. Kegel exercises, for example, involve contracting and relaxing the pelvic floor muscles in a specific pattern. This exercise can be helpful for improving urinary incontinence and other pelvic floor symptoms.

Squats are another exercise that can be helpful for strengthening the pelvic floor muscles. Squats work the glutes, quads, and hamstrings, which can help improve pelvic stability and reduce pressure on the pelvic floor. To perform a squat, stand with your feet shoulder-width apart and your toes pointing slightly outwards. Bend your knees and lower your hips down towards the ground, keeping your weight on your heels. Return to a standing position and repeat for several repetitions.

Lunges

Lunges are a popular exercise that targets several muscles, including the glutes, quads, and hamstrings. They are a versatile exercise that can be performed in a variety of ways, and their benefits extend beyond the lower body muscles they target. Below we will explore how lunges can be used to strengthen the pelvic floor muscles, improve pelvic health, and reduce the symptoms of pelvic floor dysfunction.

Pelvic floor dysfunction (PFD) is a common condition that affects many people, especially women. It refers to a group of conditions that affect the muscles, ligaments, and tissues that support the pelvic organs. PFD can lead to a range of symptoms, including urinary and fecal incontinence, pain during sex, and pelvic pain.

There are many different ways to treat PFD, and exercise is one of the most effective methods. Lunges, in particular, are a great exercise for strengthening the muscles of the pelvic floor. This is because lunges target the glutes, which are closely connected to the pelvic floor muscles. Strengthening the glutes can help to improve the function of the pelvic floor muscles and reduce symptoms of PFD.

One way that lunges can be used to strengthen the pelvic floor muscles is by incorporating them into a regular exercise routine. For example, performing lunges two to three times per week can help to build strength in the glutes and pelvic floor muscles. To perform a lunge, start by standing with your feet hip-width apart. Step forward with one foot, keeping your knee directly above your ankle. Bend your knees and lower your body until your front thigh is parallel to the ground. Then, push back up to the starting position and repeat with the other leg.

Another way to use lunges to strengthen the pelvic floor muscles is by adding resistance. This can be done by using weights or resistance bands. Adding resistance can help to increase the intensity of the exercise and provide an additional challenge for the pelvic floor muscles. When using weights or resistance bands, it is important to start with a weight that is comfortable and gradually increase the weight as you get stronger.

In addition to strengthening the pelvic floor muscles, lunges can also help to improve pelvic mobility. This is because lunges require the body to move in multiple planes of motion, which can help to increase the range of motion in the hips and pelvis. This increased mobility can help to reduce pelvic pain and discomfort, which are common symptoms of PFD.

When performing lunges, it is important to maintain proper form to avoid injury and ensure that the exercise is effective. This includes keeping your knees in line with your toes, keeping your back straight, and engaging your core muscles. It is also important to avoid arching your lower back or letting your knees collapse inward. By maintaining proper form, you can ensure that you are targeting the right muscles and getting the most out of the exercise.

Planks

Planks have become a popular exercise to strengthen the core muscles and improve overall body stability. However, planks are not just beneficial for the abs; they also have the potential to strengthen the pelvic floor muscles, making them a valuable addition to any pelvic floor exercise routine.

The pelvic floor muscles are located at the bottom of the pelvis and support the bladder, uterus, and rectum. These muscles play a crucial role in controlling urinary and bowel function, sexual function, and stability of the lower back and hips. Pelvic floor dysfunction, which can occur due to weak or tight pelvic floor muscles, can lead to a range of issues, including urinary and fecal incontinence, pelvic organ prolapse, and sexual dysfunction.

One of the main causes of weak pelvic floor muscles is lack of use or improper use. Many people unknowingly rely on other muscles to compensate for their weak pelvic floor, leading to further weakness and dysfunction. This is where exercises like planks come in.

Planks work by engaging the entire core, including the pelvic floor muscles. When done correctly, they can help improve pelvic floor strength and function. However, it is important to note that not all planks are created equal, and some variations may be more effective for pelvic floor strengthening than others.

The standard plank is performed by starting in a push-up position with the hands directly under the shoulders and the body straight from head to heels. The goal is to hold the position for as long as possible while engaging the core and keeping the hips and pelvis level. This variation can be modified to make it easier or more challenging depending on individual ability.

To make the standard plank more effective for pelvic floor strengthening, some modifications can be made. For example, instead of starting in a push-up position, begin in a forearm plank position, where the elbows are directly under the shoulders and the forearms are on the ground. This position decreases the load on the upper body and focuses more on the core and pelvic floor muscles.

Another modification that can be made is to perform a side plank. This variation targets the oblique muscles as well as the pelvic floor muscles, making it a great option for those looking to strengthen multiple areas simultaneously.

It is important to note that while planks can be an effective exercise for strengthening the pelvic floor muscles, they should not be the only exercise in a pelvic floor exercise routine. A well-rounded routine should include a variety of exercises that target different muscle groups and movements.

In addition to being an effective exercise for pelvic floor strengthening, planks offer a range of other benefits for overall health and fitness. They can help improve posture, reduce lower back pain, and increase overall body stability. Planks also require no equipment and can be done anywhere, making them a convenient exercise option for those with a busy lifestyle.

To get started with planks, it is important to start slow and gradually increase the duration and difficulty of the exercise as the pelvic floor muscles become stronger. It is also important to ensure proper form and technique to avoid injury and maximize the benefits of the exercise.

Kegel Exercises (Pelvic Floor Contractions)

- Find your pelvic floor muscles by trying to stop urine flow mid-stream (do this only to identify muscles, not as regular exercise).
- Tighten these muscles gently and hold the contraction for 5 seconds.
- Relax for 5 seconds.
- Repeat 10 times per session, 3 times a day.
- Gradually increase hold time to 10 seconds as strength improves.

2. Quick Flicks

- Contract your pelvic floor muscles quickly and tightly for 1 second.
- Release immediately.
- Repeat 10 to 20 times to improve muscle responsiveness.

3. Bridge Pose with Pelvic Floor Activation

- Lie on your back with knees bent and feet flat on the floor hip-width apart.
- Tighten your pelvic floor muscles and lift your hips off the floor, forming a straight line from shoulders to knees.

- Hold for 5 seconds, then slowly lower your hips.
- Repeat 10 times.

4. Squats with Pelvic Floor Engagement

- Stand with feet shoulder-width apart.
- As you lower into a squat, gently engage your pelvic floor muscles.
- Keep your back straight and knees behind toes.
- Return to standing while maintaining the pelvic floor contraction.
- Repeat 10 to 15 times.

5. Diaphragmatic (Deep Belly) Breathing

- Sit or lie comfortably.
- Place one hand on your belly.
- Inhale deeply through your nose, allowing your belly to rise and your pelvic floor to relax.
- Exhale slowly through your mouth while gently lifting and tightening your pelvic floor muscles.
- Repeat for 5 minutes to coordinate breath and pelvic floor movement.

6. Seated Pelvic Floor Contractions

- Sit on a chair with feet flat on the ground and back straight.

- Contract your pelvic floor muscles as if stopping urine flow.
- Hold for 5-10 seconds, then relax for the same amount of time.
- Repeat 10 times.

7. Side-Lying Pelvic Floor Activation

- Lie on your side with knees bent comfortably.
- Engage your pelvic floor muscles gently.
- Hold for 5 seconds, then relax.
- Repeat 10 times on each side.

8. Pelvic Tilts

- Lie on your back with knees bent and feet flat on the floor.
- Flatten your lower back against the floor by tightening your abdominal muscles and slightly tilting your pelvis upwards.
- At the same time, gently contract your pelvic floor muscles.
- Hold for 5 seconds, relax, and repeat 10-15 times.

9. Standing Pelvic Floor Squeezes

- While standing, contract your pelvic floor muscles for 5 seconds.
- Release and relax for 5 seconds.
- Repeat 10-15 times throughout the day during regular activities.

10. Heel Slides with Pelvic Floor Engagement

- Lie on your back with knees bent and feet flat.
- Engage your pelvic floor muscles.
- Slowly slide one heel away from your body until your leg is almost straight.
- Bring the heel back while maintaining the pelvic floor contraction.
- Repeat 10 times per leg.

Tips for Success

- Breathe normally during exercises; avoid holding your breath.
- Focus on isolating the pelvic floor muscles without tightening your abdomen, thighs, or buttocks.
- Perform exercises consistently daily for best results.
- Start slowly and increase repetitions or hold time gradually.
- If unsure about technique, consider consulting a pelvic floor physiotherapist.

Chapter Seven

Diet and Lifestyle Changes for Pelvic Floor Health

The pelvic floor is a complex system of muscles, ligaments, and nerves that support the bladder, uterus, and rectum. A strong and healthy pelvic floor is important for maintaining proper bowel and bladder function, as well as sexual health. However, many people experience pelvic floor dysfunction, which can cause a range of uncomfortable and embarrassing symptoms, such as urinary incontinence, fecal incontinence, and pelvic pain. Fortunately, there are many diet and lifestyle changes that can improve pelvic floor health and reduce the risk of pelvic floor dysfunction.

One of the most important steps to take for pelvic floor health is to maintain a healthy weight. Excess weight can put pressure on the pelvic floor muscles, causing them to weaken and lose their ability to support the pelvic organs. Losing weight through a healthy diet and exercise can help reduce this pressure and improve pelvic floor function. It's also important to avoid constipation, which can strain the pelvic floor muscles and cause them to weaken over time. Eating a diet high in fiber and staying hydrated can help prevent constipation and promote regular bowel movements.

Another key factor in pelvic floor health is regular exercise. Exercise can help strengthen the pelvic floor muscles and improve their ability to support the pelvic organs. Some exercises that are particularly beneficial for the pelvic floor include Kegels, squats, lunges, and planks. Kegels involve contracting and relaxing the pelvic floor muscles, while squats, lunges, and planks engage the entire core, including the pelvic floor. These exercises can be done at home and require no equipment, making them easy to incorporate into a daily routine.

In addition to exercise, it's important to be mindful of posture and body mechanics. Poor posture can put unnecessary strain on the pelvic floor muscles, causing them to weaken over time. Sitting up straight and avoiding slouching can help reduce this strain and improve pelvic floor function. It's also important to use proper lifting techniques, which involve engaging the pelvic floor muscles to support the weight being lifted. This can help prevent injury and reduce the risk of pelvic floor dysfunction.

Finally, reducing stress can also have a positive impact on pelvic floor health. Chronic stress can cause tension in the pelvic floor muscles, leading to pain and discomfort. Practicing stress-reducing techniques such as yoga, meditation, or deep breathing can help relax the pelvic floor muscles and improve their function.

In terms of diet, there are several foods and beverages that can have a negative impact on pelvic floor health. For example, spicy or acidic foods can irritate the bladder and cause urinary urgency or frequency. Caffeine and alcohol can also irritate the bladder and cause urinary urgency or leakage. It's best to avoid these foods and beverages or consume them in moderation to reduce the risk of pelvic floor dysfunction.

On the other hand, there are several foods and beverages that can promote pelvic floor health. Water is essential for maintaining hydration and preventing constipation, while a diet high in fiber can promote regular bowel movements and prevent straining of the pelvic floor muscles. Some studies suggest that consuming probiotics can also be beneficial for pelvic floor health, as they can help prevent urinary tract infections and promote healthy gut function.

Hydration

Hydration is a crucial component of maintaining good health, and it plays an important role in the proper functioning of the body's systems, including the pelvic floor muscles. The pelvic floor is a group of muscles that support the pelvic organs, including the bladder, uterus, and rectum. When the pelvic floor muscles are weak, individuals can experience pelvic floor dysfunction, which can lead to urinary and bowel incontinence, pelvic pain, and other problems. Below we will explore the importance of hydration in pelvic floor health and how it can help prevent or alleviate pelvic floor dysfunction.

The human body is made up of roughly 60% water, and it is essential for overall health and well-being. Adequate hydration helps to regulate body temperature, lubricate joints, flush out toxins, and transport nutrients throughout the body. In terms of the pelvic floor, hydration is crucial because it helps to keep the bladder and bowel functioning properly. When the body is dehydrated, the bladder and bowel can become constipated, which can put pressure on the pelvic floor muscles and cause them to weaken over time.

It is important to note that there is no single formula for how much water a person should drink each day. The amount of water an individual needs can vary based on their age, sex, weight, activity level, and other factors. However, a general guideline is to drink at least eight 8-ounce glasses of water per day. Additionally, it is important to drink fluids that are hydrating, such as water, herbal teas, and natural fruit juices.

One way to ensure that you are getting enough water is to monitor the color of your urine. Urine should be a pale yellow color; if it is darker, it is a sign that you are dehydrated and need to drink more fluids. Additionally, you can monitor your body weight; if you are losing weight without trying, it could be a sign that you are not drinking enough water.

In addition to staying hydrated, there are several other lifestyle changes that can help promote pelvic floor health. One of the most important things you can do is to maintain a healthy diet that is rich in fiber. This can help prevent constipation and ensure that the bowel is functioning properly. Additionally, it is important to engage in regular exercise, such as walking or yoga, to help maintain a healthy weight and strengthen the pelvic floor muscles.

It is also important to be mindful of your posture, as poor posture can put extra pressure on the pelvic floor muscles. When sitting or standing, try to keep your spine straight and your shoulders back. Avoid crossing your legs for extended periods, as this can also put pressure on the pelvic floor muscles.

In terms of hydration, it is important to be mindful of the types of fluids you are drinking. While water is the best option for staying hydrated, there are several other fluids that can be beneficial for pelvic floor health. For example, herbal teas, such as chamomile, can help reduce inflammation and promote relaxation. Cranberry juice is also beneficial, as it can help prevent urinary tract infections, which can put extra strain on the pelvic floor muscles.

High-fiber diet

A high-fiber diet is essential for good health, especially for maintaining a healthy digestive system. Fiber is found in fruits, vegetables, and whole grains and is an essential nutrient for promoting healthy digestion, regular bowel movements, and maintaining the overall health of the body. A high-fiber diet can also be beneficial for individuals with pelvic floor dysfunction.

Pelvic floor dysfunction is a common condition where the muscles and connective tissues in the pelvic region become weakened or damaged, leading to problems with bladder and bowel control, pelvic pain, and sexual dysfunction. There are many factors that can contribute to the development of pelvic floor dysfunction, including pregnancy, childbirth, aging, and chronic constipation. However, diet and lifestyle factors can also play a role.

One of the most effective ways to improve pelvic floor health is through dietary changes, including the inclusion of high-fiber foods. High-fiber foods help to regulate bowel movements and reduce constipation, which can put extra strain on the pelvic floor muscles. In addition, a high-fiber diet can help to promote the growth of healthy gut bacteria, which can have a positive impact on overall gut health.

There are two types of fiber, soluble and insoluble. Soluble fiber dissolves in water and forms a gel-like substance, which helps to slow down the passage of food through the digestive system. Insoluble fiber does not dissolve in water and adds bulk to the stool, which helps to promote regular bowel movements. Both types of fiber are important for maintaining good health.

Good sources of soluble fiber include fruits, vegetables, legumes, oats, and flaxseeds. These foods help to promote the growth of healthy gut bacteria, which can have a positive impact on overall digestive health. Insoluble fiber is found in whole grains, nuts, seeds, and vegetables like broccoli and carrots. These foods help to add bulk to the stool, which can help to prevent constipation and reduce the strain on the pelvic floor muscles.

In addition to including high-fiber foods in the diet, it is also important to drink plenty of fluids. Adequate hydration helps to keep the stool soft and easy to pass, reducing the strain on the pelvic floor muscles. Drinking plenty of water and other fluids also helps to promote healthy kidney function, which is important for overall health and well-being.

It is important to note that sudden increases in fiber intake can cause digestive discomfort, including bloating, gas, and diarrhea. It is recommended that individuals gradually increase their fiber intake over several weeks to allow the digestive system to adjust. In addition, it is important to drink plenty of fluids when increasing fiber intake to help prevent constipation.

In addition to dietary changes, there are several lifestyle factors that can contribute to pelvic floor health. Exercise is an important component of pelvic floor health, and regular physical activity can help to improve muscle tone and reduce the risk of pelvic floor dysfunction. Certain types of exercise, such as yoga and Pilates, can be particularly beneficial for pelvic floor health, as they focus on strengthening the core muscles that support the pelvic floor.

Maintaining a healthy weight is also important for pelvic floor health. Excess weight can put extra strain on the pelvic floor muscles, leading to weakening and damage over time. A healthy diet and regular exercise can help to maintain a healthy weight and reduce the risk of pelvic floor dysfunction.

Avoiding irritants (caffeine, alcohol, acidic foods)

Pelvic floor dysfunction is a common condition that affects many people, particularly women. It is characterized by weakness, tightness, or dysfunction of the muscles that support the pelvic organs, including the bladder, uterus, and rectum. This can lead to a range of symptoms, including urinary incontinence, pelvic pain, and constipation. While there are many treatment options available for pelvic floor dysfunction, one effective strategy is making dietary and lifestyle changes to support pelvic floor health.

One important dietary change that can support pelvic floor health is avoiding irritants such as caffeine, alcohol, and acidic foods. Caffeine, found in coffee, tea, and many sodas, is a diuretic that can cause increased urinary frequency and urgency, which can exacerbate symptoms of urinary incontinence. Alcohol can also irritate the bladder and lead to increased urinary frequency, as well as constipation. Acidic foods, such as citrus fruits and tomatoes, can irritate the bladder and contribute to symptoms of urinary urgency and pain.

In addition to avoiding irritants, it is important to maintain a healthy and balanced diet to support pelvic floor health. One key component of a healthy diet is fiber, which helps to regulate bowel movements and prevent constipation. Constipation can put strain on the pelvic floor muscles, leading to weakness and dysfunction over time. A high-fiber diet can also help to prevent hemorrhoids, which can be a painful and uncomfortable complication of pelvic floor dysfunction.

Hydration is another important aspect of maintaining pelvic floor health. Drinking plenty of water and other fluids can help to keep the bladder and bowels functioning properly and prevent constipation. Dehydration can contribute to urinary tract infections, which can worsen symptoms of pelvic floor dysfunction. It is important to aim for at least eight glasses of water per day, and more if you are exercising or in hot weather.

Exercise is also important for maintaining pelvic floor health, but it is important to choose exercises that are gentle and low-impact to avoid exacerbating symptoms of pelvic floor dysfunction. Yoga and Pilates are two types of exercise that are particularly beneficial for the pelvic floor muscles, as they focus on core strength and stability. Kegel exercises, which involve contracting and relaxing the muscles of the pelvic floor, can also be a helpful way to strengthen these muscles and improve symptoms of urinary incontinence.

In addition to these dietary and lifestyle changes, there are other strategies that can be used to manage pelvic floor dysfunction. Pelvic floor physical therapy, which involves working with a trained therapist to strengthen and relax the muscles of the pelvic floor, can be an effective treatment option. Biofeedback, which uses sensors to help individuals learn how to control and strengthen their pelvic floor muscles, can also be helpful. In some cases, surgery may be necessary to correct structural issues that are contributing to pelvic floor dysfunction.

Maintaining a healthy weight

Maintaining a healthy weight is essential for overall health and wellbeing, and it can also have a significant impact on pelvic floor health. The pelvic floor muscles play a crucial role in supporting the bladder, uterus, and rectum. When these muscles become weak or damaged, it can lead to pelvic floor dysfunction, including urinary incontinence, fecal incontinence, and pelvic organ prolapse. Maintaining a healthy weight through proper diet and exercise can help reduce the risk of developing pelvic floor dysfunction.

Carrying excess weight can put added pressure on the pelvic floor muscles, causing them to weaken over time. This pressure can also increase the risk of pelvic organ prolapse, which occurs when the organs in the pelvic area, such as the bladder or uterus, drop from their normal position and push against the vaginal walls. Women who are overweight or obese are at a higher risk of developing pelvic organ prolapse, especially after menopause.

In addition to the physical strain on the pelvic floor muscles, excess weight can also increase the risk of developing chronic conditions such as diabetes and heart disease. These conditions can further contribute to pelvic floor dysfunction and weaken the muscles over time.

Fortunately, making lifestyle changes to maintain a healthy weight can help reduce the risk of developing pelvic floor dysfunction. The first step is to ensure that your diet is well-balanced and includes a variety of nutrient-dense foods. Eating a diet that is high in fruits, vegetables, whole grains, and lean protein sources can help maintain a healthy weight and reduce the risk of chronic conditions.

It is also important to limit your intake of highly processed and sugary foods, as well as foods that are high in saturated and trans fats. These types of foods can contribute to inflammation and weight gain, both of which can negatively impact pelvic floor health.

In addition to a healthy diet, regular exercise can also help maintain a healthy weight and reduce the risk of pelvic floor dysfunction. Exercise can help strengthen the pelvic floor muscles, as well as improve overall muscle tone and flexibility. Engaging in regular physical activity can also help reduce stress and improve sleep, both of which can contribute to a healthy weight and overall health.

However, it is important to note that certain types of exercises can put excessive strain on the pelvic floor muscles and should be avoided or modified. High-impact exercises such as running, jumping, or heavy lifting can put pressure on the pelvic floor and contribute to pelvic floor dysfunction. Instead, low-impact exercises such as walking, cycling, swimming, or yoga can be effective ways to maintain a healthy weight and improve pelvic floor health without causing additional strain.

It is also important to maintain proper form during exercises to avoid putting unnecessary pressure on the pelvic floor muscles. Engaging in exercises that strengthen the core muscles, such as planks or bridges, can help improve overall muscle tone and reduce the risk of pelvic floor dysfunction.

In addition to maintaining a healthy weight through diet and exercise, other lifestyle factors can also impact pelvic floor health. For example, smoking can weaken the pelvic floor muscles and increase the risk of chronic conditions such as heart disease and cancer, which can further contribute to pelvic floor dysfunction. It is important to avoid smoking and exposure to secondhand smoke to maintain pelvic floor health.

Avoiding constipation

Avoiding Constipation: Tips for a Healthy Pelvic Floor

The pelvic floor muscles play an important role in the body, supporting the bladder, uterus, and rectum. However, many people are unaware of how important it is to maintain a healthy pelvic floor, and how certain lifestyle factors can affect it. One of these factors is constipation, which can put a strain on the pelvic floor and contribute to pelvic floor dysfunction. Below we will discuss what constipation is, how it affects the pelvic floor, and some tips for avoiding it to maintain a healthy pelvic floor.

What is Constipation?

Constipation is a common digestive problem where a person has difficulty passing stools, or has infrequent bowel movements. It can be caused by a variety of factors, including a lack of fiber in the diet, dehydration, medication side effects, and a sedentary lifestyle. Constipation can lead to discomfort, bloating, and abdominal pain, and if left untreated, it can cause long-term damage to the colon.

How Does Constipation Affect the Pelvic Floor?

When a person is constipated, they may strain to pass stools. This straining can put pressure on the pelvic floor muscles, which can lead to weakness or damage over time. Additionally, chronic constipation can cause the muscles of the pelvic floor to become stretched and weakened, leading to issues such as urinary incontinence and pelvic organ prolapse.

Tips for Avoiding Constipation

The good news is that constipation can often be prevented with some simple lifestyle changes. Here are some tips for maintaining a healthy digestive system and avoiding constipation:

Eat a High-Fiber Diet

One of the most important factors in preventing constipation is getting enough fiber in the diet. Fiber helps to keep the stool soft and bulky, which makes it easier to pass. Good sources of fiber include whole grains, fruits, vegetables, and legumes. It's important to gradually increase fiber intake to avoid bloating and discomfort.

Drink Plenty of Water

Dehydration can make constipation worse, so it's important to drink plenty of water throughout the day. Experts recommend drinking at least eight glasses of water per day, but this can vary depending on individual needs.

Exercise Regularly

Physical activity can help to stimulate the digestive system and promote regular bowel movements. Even a simple 30-minute walk each day can be beneficial. Exercise also strengthens the muscles of the pelvic floor, which can help to prevent pelvic floor dysfunction.

Avoid Irritants

Certain foods and drinks can irritate the digestive system and contribute to constipation. These include caffeine, alcohol, and acidic foods such as tomatoes and citrus fruits. It's important to be mindful of these irritants and limit them in the diet.

Practice Good Bathroom Habits

When using the bathroom, it's important to take the time to fully empty the bowels. Straining or rushing can put unnecessary pressure on the pelvic floor muscles. It's also important to use the correct posture on the toilet - sitting with the feet on a small stool can help to promote better bowel movements.

Manage Stress

Stress can have a negative impact on the digestive system and contribute to constipation. Finding healthy ways to manage stress, such as through exercise, relaxation techniques, or therapy, can help to promote better digestive health.

Chapter Eight

Strategies for Coping with Pelvic Floor Disorders

Pelvic floor disorders can significantly impact a person's quality of life, causing a range of uncomfortable symptoms like urinary incontinence, fecal incontinence, pelvic pain, and sexual dysfunction. While there are several treatments available for pelvic floor disorders, including medication, surgery, and physical therapy, there are also many strategies that people can use to cope with the condition on a day-to-day basis. Below we will discuss some of these strategies and how they can help people manage the symptoms of pelvic floor disorders.

Mind-Body Techniques

Stress can exacerbate the symptoms of pelvic floor disorders. That's why mind-body techniques like yoga, meditation, and deep breathing exercises can be effective in managing the condition. These techniques can help reduce stress levels, which in turn can reduce muscle tension in the pelvic floor region. This can help alleviate symptoms like pain and discomfort.

Pelvic Floor Muscle Exercises

Pelvic floor muscle exercises, also known as Kegels, can be beneficial for people with pelvic floor disorders. These exercises can help strengthen the muscles that support the pelvic organs, which can help reduce urinary and fecal incontinence, as well as improve sexual function. It's important to do these exercises correctly, and a physical therapist can provide guidance on how to perform them effectively.

Diet Modification

Certain foods and drinks can irritate the bladder and worsen the symptoms of pelvic floor disorders. Some common irritants include caffeine, alcohol, spicy foods, and acidic foods. Avoiding these foods or limiting their intake can help reduce symptoms. It's also important to stay hydrated and maintain a healthy diet rich in fiber, as constipation can exacerbate symptoms.

Bladder and Bowel Habits

People with pelvic floor disorders should pay attention to their bladder and bowel habits. This means going to the bathroom when you need to and not holding in urine or feces for extended periods. It's also important to empty the bladder completely and take your time when using the toilet, as rushing can lead to incomplete voiding. Additionally, if constipation is an issue, you may need to establish a regular bowel routine and consider the use of stool softeners or laxatives.

Pessaries

A pessary is a device that is inserted into the vagina to help support the pelvic organs. Pessaries come in different shapes and sizes, and they can be a helpful tool for people with pelvic floor disorders. A healthcare provider can help determine which type of pessary is best suited for your needs.

Clothing Choices

Wearing tight clothing can put pressure on the pelvic floor muscles, which can worsen symptoms. Opting for loose-fitting clothing made of breathable fabrics can help reduce discomfort and pain associated with pelvic floor disorders.

Physical Therapy

Physical therapy can be an effective treatment for pelvic floor disorders. A physical therapist can provide guidance on pelvic floor muscle exercises, as well as other exercises that can help improve pelvic floor function. They can also provide education on proper bladder and bowel habits and help with the use of devices like pessaries.

Emotional Support

Living with a pelvic floor disorder can be challenging, and it's important to seek emotional support if needed. Talking to a counselor or joining a support group can provide a safe space to discuss your experiences, as well as help you learn coping strategies and connect with others who are going through similar experiences.

Pelvic floor physical therapy

Pelvic floor dysfunction is a common problem among women, especially after childbirth, but it can also occur in men. The pelvic floor muscles are responsible for supporting the bladder, uterus, and rectum, as well as controlling urination and bowel movements. When these muscles weaken or become damaged, it can result in a variety of symptoms such as incontinence, painful intercourse, and pelvic pain. Pelvic floor physical therapy is a specialized type of therapy that can help improve the strength and function of these muscles. Below we will discuss the benefits of pelvic floor physical therapy and how it can help people cope with pelvic floor disorders.

Pelvic floor physical therapy is a specialized type of physical therapy that focuses on the muscles, ligaments, and connective tissues that support the pelvic organs. The goal of pelvic floor physical therapy is to help people regain control of their pelvic muscles and reduce symptoms of pelvic floor dysfunction. This type of therapy can be performed by a trained physical therapist who has specialized training in pelvic floor disorders.

One of the main benefits of pelvic floor physical therapy is that it is non-invasive and does not involve any medications or surgery. This makes it a safe and effective option for people who want to avoid more invasive treatments. During a pelvic floor physical therapy session, the therapist will assess the patient's pelvic floor muscles and develop a treatment plan tailored to their specific needs.

There are many different techniques that can be used during pelvic floor physical therapy, including exercises, manual therapy, biofeedback, and electrical stimulation. Exercises are often used to help strengthen the pelvic floor muscles and improve their function. Manual therapy involves the therapist using their hands to massage or stretch the pelvic floor muscles. Biofeedback is a technique that uses sensors to measure the activity of the pelvic floor muscles and provide feedback to the patient. Electrical stimulation involves using a small electrical current to stimulate the pelvic floor muscles and improve their function.

Pelvic floor physical therapy can be beneficial for a variety of pelvic floor disorders, including urinary incontinence, fecal incontinence, pelvic pain, and painful intercourse. Studies have shown that pelvic floor physical therapy can improve symptoms of urinary incontinence in women by up to 75%. It has also been shown to be effective in treating fecal incontinence, with up to 70% of patients experiencing improvement in their symptoms.

In addition to improving symptoms of pelvic floor dysfunction, pelvic floor physical therapy can also help prevent these problems from occurring in the first place. For example, pelvic floor exercises can help strengthen the pelvic floor muscles during pregnancy, which can reduce the risk of developing urinary incontinence after childbirth.

It is important to note that pelvic floor physical therapy may not be effective for everyone with pelvic floor dysfunction. In some cases, surgery or medication may be necessary to treat the underlying problem. However, for many people, pelvic floor physical therapy can be a safe and effective way to improve the strength and function of their pelvic floor muscles.

Support groups

Support groups are an excellent way for individuals with pelvic floor dysfunction to connect with others who have similar experiences. These groups provide a safe and supportive environment where members can share their struggles, learn from one another, and receive emotional support.

Pelvic floor dysfunction refers to a group of conditions that affect the pelvic floor muscles, which are responsible for controlling bowel and bladder function, as well as sexual activity. This can lead to a range of symptoms, including pain or discomfort in the pelvic region, urinary and/or fecal incontinence, and difficulty achieving orgasm.

For many people, living with pelvic floor dysfunction can be isolating, frustrating, and even embarrassing. However, joining a support group can help to alleviate some of these feelings by providing a space where individuals can connect with others who understand what they are going through.

One of the main benefits of support groups is that they allow individuals to share their experiences and emotions with others who are going through similar struggles. This can be a great source of comfort and validation, as members can offer each other advice, encouragement, and support. Knowing that others are going through similar experiences can also help individuals feel less alone in their journey.

In addition to emotional support, support groups can also provide practical advice and information. Many groups invite experts to speak on topics such as pelvic floor exercises, medical treatments, and lifestyle modifications. Members can also share their own strategies for managing symptoms and improving their quality of life.

Support groups can take many forms, from in-person meetings to online communities. In-person groups typically meet on a regular basis, such as once a month, and provide an opportunity for members to connect face-to-face. Online groups, on the other hand, allow individuals to connect from the comfort of their own home and offer the flexibility of being able to participate at any time of day or night.

It is important to note that while support groups can be a valuable resource for individuals with pelvic floor dysfunction, they are not a substitute for professional medical care. It is important for individuals to work with their healthcare provider to develop a treatment plan that meets their specific needs.

To find a support group, individuals can start by asking their healthcare provider for recommendations. They can also search online for local support groups or online communities. Many advocacy organizations also offer support groups for individuals with specific conditions, such as interstitial cystitis or endometriosis.

In addition to joining a support group, there are other strategies individuals can use to cope with pelvic floor dysfunction. These may include practicing relaxation techniques, such as deep breathing or meditation, staying active and engaging in regular exercise, and developing a self-care routine that prioritizes physical and emotional well-being.

Mental health counselling

Mental health is an essential aspect of overall well-being, and it plays a crucial role in the management of various health conditions, including pelvic floor dysfunction. Pelvic floor dysfunction refers to a group of conditions that affect the muscles, ligaments, and nerves that support the pelvic organs, including the bladder, uterus, and rectum. Symptoms of pelvic floor dysfunction may include pain or discomfort in the pelvic region, urinary or bowel problems, and sexual dysfunction. These symptoms can have a significant impact on an individual's mental health, leading to anxiety, depression, and other psychological issues. Below we will explore the role of mental health counselling in the management of pelvic floor dysfunction.

The relationship between mental health and pelvic floor dysfunction is complex and multi-faceted. Pelvic floor dysfunction can cause significant physical discomfort, leading to anxiety and stress. These emotional responses can exacerbate the symptoms of pelvic floor dysfunction, creating a vicious cycle of pain, anxiety, and stress. Additionally, pelvic floor dysfunction can have a significant impact on an individual's quality of life, affecting their ability to engage in daily activities, work, and social interactions. These changes can lead to feelings of isolation, shame, and embarrassment, further impacting mental health.

Mental health counselling is an effective approach to managing the psychological aspects of pelvic floor dysfunction. A mental health counselor can provide emotional support, help individuals understand and manage their emotions, and develop coping strategies to deal with the physical symptoms of pelvic floor dysfunction. Mental health counselling can also help individuals to identify and address any underlying psychological issues that may be contributing to their symptoms, such as anxiety or depression.

There are several types of mental health counselling approaches that can be used to manage the psychological aspects of pelvic floor dysfunction. One common approach is cognitive-behavioral therapy (CBT). CBT is a short-term, goal-oriented therapy that focuses on changing negative patterns of thought and behavior. This therapy can help individuals identify and modify negative thoughts and behaviors that may be contributing to their pelvic floor dysfunction symptoms. For example, a therapist may work with an individual to identify any fears or anxieties they may have about engaging in sexual activity, and help them develop strategies to overcome these fears.

Another type of mental health counselling approach that may be used in the management of pelvic floor dysfunction is mindfulness-based therapy. Mindfulness-based therapy involves the practice of mindfulness meditation, which can help individuals become more aware of their thoughts and emotions. This therapy can help individuals develop a greater sense of control over their emotions, leading to reduced stress and anxiety levels. Mindfulness-based therapy can also be helpful in managing chronic pain, which is a common symptom of pelvic floor dysfunction.

Pelvic floor dysfunction can also have a significant impact on an individual's relationship with their partner. This can lead to feelings of isolation and loneliness, which can further exacerbate mental health issues. Couple's therapy may be a useful approach to managing the psychological aspects of pelvic floor dysfunction. This therapy can help partners improve their communication skills, understand each other's needs and concerns, and develop strategies to improve intimacy and sexual function.

In addition to mental health counselling, there are several self-care strategies that individuals with pelvic floor dysfunction can use to manage their mental health. These strategies may include regular exercise, relaxation techniques such as deep breathing or meditation, and engaging in activities that bring joy and fulfillment, such as hobbies or social activities.

What is the prognosis for Pelvic Floor Disorder

Pelvic floor disorders refer to a range of conditions that affect the muscles, ligaments, and connective tissues that support the pelvic organs. These disorders can be caused by pregnancy, childbirth, aging, obesity, surgery, and other medical conditions. Symptoms of pelvic floor disorders can include urinary and fecal incontinence, pelvic pain, and sexual dysfunction. Many people with pelvic floor disorders are curious about their prognosis, or the likely course and outcome of their condition.

Prognosis for pelvic floor disorders can vary widely depending on the specific disorder, its severity, and the underlying cause. Some pelvic floor disorders can be cured or significantly improved with proper treatment, while others may be chronic and require long-term management. In general, early diagnosis and treatment can improve the prognosis for pelvic floor disorders.

Urinary incontinence is a common pelvic floor disorder, affecting up to one-third of women and one-fifth of men. The prognosis for urinary incontinence depends on the underlying cause and severity of the condition. For example, stress incontinence, which is caused by weakened pelvic floor muscles, can often be improved with pelvic floor muscle exercises, lifestyle modifications, and other non-surgical treatments. However, some cases of urinary incontinence may require surgery or other more invasive treatments. Overall, the prognosis for urinary incontinence is generally good with proper treatment.

Fecal incontinence is another common pelvic floor disorder, affecting up to 15% of adults. The prognosis for fecal incontinence depends on the underlying cause and severity of the condition. For example, mild cases of fecal incontinence may be improved with pelvic floor muscle exercises, dietary modifications, and medications. However, more severe cases may require surgery or other more invasive treatments. The prognosis for fecal incontinence can be good with proper treatment, but the condition can be chronic and require ongoing management.

Pelvic organ prolapse is a pelvic floor disorder that occurs when the muscles and tissues that support the pelvic organs become weak or damaged, causing the organs to bulge into the vaginal wall or protrude outside the body. The prognosis for pelvic organ prolapse depends on the severity of the condition and the underlying cause. Mild cases of pelvic organ prolapse may be managed with pelvic floor muscle exercises and other non-surgical treatments, while more severe cases may require surgery. The prognosis for pelvic organ prolapse can be good with proper treatment, but the condition can recur even after successful treatment.

Pelvic pain is a common symptom of pelvic floor disorders, and can be caused by a variety of underlying conditions such as endometriosis, interstitial cystitis, and pelvic floor muscle dysfunction. The prognosis for pelvic pain depends on the underlying cause and severity of the condition. Some cases of pelvic pain may be improved with physical therapy, medications, and other non-surgical treatments. However, more severe cases may require surgery or other more invasive treatments. The prognosis for pelvic pain can be good with proper treatment, but the condition can be chronic and require ongoing management.

Sexual dysfunction is another common symptom of pelvic floor disorders, and can be caused by a variety of underlying conditions such as vaginal atrophy, pelvic organ prolapse, and vulvodynia. The prognosis for sexual dysfunction depends on the underlying cause and severity of the condition. Some cases of sexual dysfunction may be improved with physical therapy, medications, and other non-surgical treatments. However, more severe cases may require surgery or other more invasive treatments. The prognosis for sexual dysfunction can be good with proper treatment, but the condition can be chronic and require ongoing management.

Chapter Nine

Coping with a Pelvic Floor Disorder

Coping with a pelvic floor disorder can be challenging, but there are strategies that can help individuals manage their symptoms and improve their quality of life. Pelvic floor disorders refer to a group of conditions that affect the muscles, ligaments, and connective tissues in the pelvic region, including the bladder, uterus, rectum, and vagina. These conditions can cause a range of symptoms, including urinary or fecal incontinence, pain during sexual intercourse, and pelvic pain.

The first step in coping with a pelvic floor disorder is to seek medical attention. A healthcare provider can help diagnose the specific condition and recommend treatment options. Treatment may include pelvic floor exercises, medication, or surgery, depending on the severity of the condition.

In addition to medical treatment, there are several strategies that can help individuals cope with pelvic floor disorders. One of the most effective strategies is pelvic floor physical therapy. This type of therapy involves working with a trained therapist to strengthen and stretch the pelvic floor muscles. The therapist may also use techniques such as biofeedback or electrical stimulation to help individuals learn how to properly contract and relax the pelvic floor muscles.

Another strategy for coping with pelvic floor disorders is maintaining a healthy lifestyle. This includes eating a balanced diet, staying hydrated, and getting regular exercise. A high-fiber diet can help prevent constipation, which is a common cause of pelvic floor disorders. Similarly, staying hydrated can help prevent constipation and reduce the risk of urinary tract infections.

Regular exercise can also help strengthen the pelvic floor muscles and reduce symptoms of pelvic floor disorders. However, it is important to choose exercises that do not put too much pressure on the pelvic floor, such as walking, swimming, or cycling. High-impact exercises such as running or jumping can actually make symptoms worse.

In addition to physical strategies, it is important to address the emotional impact of pelvic floor disorders. Living with a chronic condition can be stressful and can lead to anxiety or depression. Seeking support from friends, family, or a support group can help individuals feel less alone and better able to cope with their condition.

Mental health counseling can also be helpful in managing the emotional impact of pelvic floor disorders. A counselor can help individuals develop coping strategies for managing stress, anxiety, or depression related to their condition. In some cases, medication may also be recommended to help manage symptoms of anxiety or depression.

Finally, it is important to remember that coping with a pelvic floor disorder is an ongoing process. It may take time to find the right treatment approach, and individuals may need to adjust their strategies over time as their condition changes. However, with the right treatment and support, it is possible to manage symptoms and improve quality of life.

Emotional impact of a Disorder Pelvic Floor

The pelvic floor is a complex network of muscles, ligaments, and nerves that work together to support the bladder, uterus, and rectum. Pelvic floor dysfunction (PFD) is a common condition that affects both men and women and can lead to a wide range of symptoms, including incontinence, constipation, pain, and sexual dysfunction. While the physical effects of PFD can be challenging to manage, it's important not to overlook the emotional impact of the condition.

People with PFD may experience a range of emotions, including anxiety, depression, embarrassment, frustration, and isolation. Living with PFD can be overwhelming, especially if the symptoms are severe or affect your quality of life. It can be challenging to talk about PFD with friends, family, or even healthcare providers, which can lead to feelings of shame and isolation.

The emotional impact of PFD is often underestimated and can have a significant impact on a person's mental health and wellbeing. Many people with PFD experience anxiety and depression, which can exacerbate their symptoms and make it harder to manage the condition. For example, anxiety can cause muscle tension, which can worsen PFD symptoms. Depression can make it challenging to maintain a healthy lifestyle, including regular exercise and a balanced diet, which are essential for managing PFD symptoms.

People with PFD may also experience embarrassment and shame about their condition. Incontinence, for example, can be challenging to manage and can lead to embarrassing situations, such as leaking urine in public. This can lead to feelings of shame and can cause people to avoid social situations, which can further isolate them from their friends and family.

The emotional impact of PFD can also affect sexual health and intimacy. Many people with PFD experience pain during sex or may find it difficult to achieve or maintain an erection or orgasm. These symptoms can be frustrating and may cause people to avoid sexual activity altogether, which can put a strain on their relationships.

Despite the challenges of living with PFD, there are strategies that can help people cope with the emotional impact of the condition. One important step is to seek emotional support from friends, family, or a mental health professional. Talking about your feelings and concerns can help you feel less isolated and more empowered to manage your symptoms.

Exercise can also be an effective way to manage the emotional impact of PFD. Regular exercise has been shown to reduce anxiety and depression and can also help strengthen the pelvic floor muscles. There are many exercises that can help strengthen the pelvic floor, including Kegels, squats, and yoga.

In addition to exercise, maintaining a healthy lifestyle can also help manage the emotional impact of PFD. Eating a balanced diet, getting enough sleep, and avoiding alcohol and caffeine can all help reduce anxiety and depression and improve overall health and wellbeing.

Finally, joining a support group can be an effective way to connect with other people who are living with PFD. Support groups provide a safe and supportive environment where people can share their experiences, ask questions, and get advice from others who have gone through similar experiences. Support groups can also help reduce feelings of isolation and provide a sense of community and belonging.

Coping strategies for patients and caregivers

Coping with a chronic condition like pelvic floor dysfunction (PFD) can be challenging, not just for patients but also for their caregivers. PFD refers to a variety of conditions that affect the muscles, nerves, and connective tissue that support the pelvic organs, including the bladder, uterus, rectum, and prostate. Symptoms of PFD can range from urinary or fecal incontinence, painful sex, to chronic pelvic pain. Coping strategies are essential for PFD patients and their caregivers to manage the emotional, physical, and practical challenges that come with the condition.

One of the essential coping strategies for PFD patients and caregivers is education. Knowledge about the condition, its symptoms, causes, and treatment options can be empowering, reduce anxiety and improve the quality of life. Understanding the condition can help patients and caregivers develop realistic expectations and make informed decisions about their care. They can learn about pelvic floor exercises, diet, and lifestyle modifications that can help manage the symptoms.

Pelvic floor physical therapy is another essential coping strategy for PFD patients. A physical therapist can teach patients how to do pelvic floor exercises, which can help strengthen the pelvic muscles and reduce urinary and fecal incontinence, as well as pain. Pelvic floor physical therapy can also help reduce pain during intercourse, improve sexual function, and improve quality of life.

Counseling can also be an essential coping strategy for PFD patients and caregivers. A diagnosis of PFD can be distressing, and many patients and caregivers may experience anxiety, depression, and other emotional challenges. Counseling can provide a safe space to express emotions, work through challenges, and develop coping skills. It can also help patients and caregivers communicate more effectively with their healthcare providers and manage their care more effectively.

Support groups can also be a valuable coping strategy for PFD patients and caregivers. Support groups provide a safe and supportive environment where patients and caregivers can share their experiences, learn from each other, and provide emotional support. Support groups can also be a valuable source of information and practical advice about managing PFD. There are many online and in-person support groups available, and patients and caregivers can ask their healthcare provider for recommendations.

Practical coping strategies are also essential for PFD patients and caregivers. Patients may need to make modifications to their lifestyle, such as reducing caffeine intake, maintaining a healthy weight, and avoiding constipation. Caregivers may need to help patients manage their symptoms, such as assisting with toileting or helping patients perform pelvic floor exercises. Practical coping strategies can also include making modifications to the home environment, such as installing grab bars or raised toilet seats.

The role of diet in Pelvic Floor Disorders

Pelvic Floor Disorders (PFD) affect millions of people worldwide and can significantly impact a person's quality of life. While there are many treatments available, one often overlooked aspect of PFD is the role of diet. Diet plays a crucial role in the development and management of PFD. Below we will discuss the role of diet in PFD and how dietary changes can help manage PFD.

The pelvic floor is a group of muscles, ligaments, and connective tissue that support the pelvic organs, including the bladder, uterus, and rectum. When these muscles weaken or become damaged, it can lead to a range of symptoms, including urinary incontinence, bowel incontinence, pelvic pain, and sexual dysfunction.

Dietary factors play a role in the development and management of PFD. Certain foods and drinks can irritate the bladder and bowel, leading to symptoms like urinary urgency, frequency, and incontinence, as well as constipation and fecal incontinence. Therefore, it is essential to make dietary changes to manage PFD.

Foods that can irritate the bladder include acidic foods and drinks like citrus fruits, tomatoes, vinegar, and carbonated beverages. Caffeine and alcohol are also known irritants that can lead to bladder irritation and exacerbate symptoms like urinary urgency and frequency. It is best to limit these foods and drinks or avoid them altogether.

Fiber-rich foods are essential for maintaining good bowel health. They help prevent constipation and promote regular bowel movements. However, certain high-fiber foods, like beans, can cause gas and bloating, which can aggravate PFD symptoms. Therefore, it is important to consume fiber-rich foods in moderation and gradually increase fiber intake to avoid gastrointestinal distress.

Another essential aspect of diet in managing PFD is maintaining a healthy weight. Being overweight or obese can put additional pressure on the pelvic floor muscles, leading to weakening and damage. Therefore, it is essential to maintain a healthy weight through a balanced diet and regular exercise.

In addition to dietary changes, it is also essential to stay hydrated. Dehydration can lead to constipation, which can exacerbate PFD symptoms. Drinking plenty of water and other fluids can help keep bowel movements regular and prevent constipation.

Finally, it is important to note that dietary changes alone may not be enough to manage PFD. A comprehensive treatment plan that includes pelvic floor physical therapy, medication, and surgery may be necessary depending on the severity of the condition. However, dietary changes can be an effective adjunct therapy to manage symptoms and improve overall pelvic floor health.

The role of stress in Pelvic Floor Disorders

Pelvic Floor Disorders (PFD) are a common health problem that affects millions of people worldwide. It can cause various symptoms, such as pelvic pain, urinary and fecal incontinence, and sexual dysfunction. While many factors can contribute to the development of PFD, stress is one that is often overlooked. Below we will explore the role of stress in Pelvic Floor Disorders and how it can affect the pelvic floor muscles.

Stress is a normal part of life, and the body has a natural response to it. When we experience stress, the body releases hormones such as adrenaline and cortisol, which prepare us to respond to the stressor. However, chronic stress can cause a range of health problems, including PFD. When stress becomes chronic, the body remains in a constant state of alert, which can cause tension and tightness in the pelvic floor muscles.

One of the most common pelvic floor disorders associated with stress is pelvic pain. Chronic stress can cause the pelvic floor muscles to become tight and hypertonic, leading to pain and discomfort in the pelvic region. This pain can be exacerbated by physical activity, sitting for long periods, or sexual intercourse. Women who have experienced trauma or abuse, which can lead to chronic stress, are particularly vulnerable to developing pelvic pain.

Stress can also contribute to urinary and fecal incontinence. When we are stressed, we tend to hold tension in our pelvic floor muscles, which can weaken them over time. Weak pelvic floor muscles can lead to urinary and fecal incontinence, as the muscles are unable to contract effectively to control the bladder and bowel. This can be particularly problematic for women during pregnancy and after childbirth when the pelvic floor muscles are already weakened.

Sexual dysfunction is another common symptom of PFD that can be exacerbated by stress. When we are stressed, our bodies produce less estrogen and testosterone, which can decrease our libido and make it difficult to become aroused. Chronic stress can also cause tension in the pelvic floor muscles, making it difficult to achieve orgasm.

So, what can be done to manage the impact of stress on Pelvic Floor Disorders? Firstly, it is important to identify and manage the sources of stress in your life. This may involve making lifestyle changes such as reducing your workload or increasing your exercise routine. Secondly, relaxation techniques such as deep breathing, meditation, and yoga can help to reduce tension in the pelvic floor muscles and promote overall relaxation. This can be particularly helpful for women who have experienced trauma or abuse, as these techniques can help to release emotional tension stored in the body.

Pelvic Floor Physical Therapy (PFPT) can also be an effective treatment for PFD caused by stress. PFPT involves working with a physical therapist who specializes in pelvic floor disorders to learn exercises that can help to strengthen and relax the pelvic floor muscles. These exercises can be particularly helpful for women who have weak or hypertonic pelvic floor muscles, which can lead to pelvic pain, incontinence, and sexual dysfunction.

What are the risks and complications associated with a Pelvic Floor Disorder

Pelvic floor disorders are a common health problem affecting millions of people worldwide, with symptoms ranging from mild to severe. These disorders are often associated with several risks and complications, which may significantly impact a person's quality of life. Below we will explore the various risks and complications associated with pelvic floor disorders.

One of the most common risks associated with pelvic floor disorders is urinary incontinence. This condition causes an individual to lose control over their bladder, resulting in unintentional urine leakage. This can be particularly embarrassing and distressing, leading to social isolation and depression.

Another risk associated with pelvic floor disorders is fecal incontinence, which causes an individual to lose control over their bowel movements. This can result in severe social stigma and can impact a person's quality of life, leading to anxiety and depression.

Pelvic floor disorders can also cause pelvic pain, which can be chronic and debilitating. This pain may be due to the muscles of the pelvic floor being in a constant state of tension, resulting in discomfort and difficulty with activities such as sitting, standing, and walking.

Furthermore, pelvic floor disorders can cause sexual dysfunction, including pain during intercourse, difficulty achieving or maintaining an erection, or difficulty achieving orgasm. These complications can significantly impact a person's self-esteem and quality of life, leading to depression and anxiety.

Aside from these physical complications, pelvic floor disorders can also impact an individual's mental health. Chronic pelvic pain can lead to depression and anxiety, with patients often reporting a sense of isolation and hopelessness. Additionally, the fear of embarrassing symptoms, such as incontinence, can cause significant stress and anxiety, leading to a decline in overall quality of life.

The complications of pelvic floor disorders can have a significant impact on a person's daily life. It can result in social isolation, depression, anxiety, and a reduced quality of life. However, it is essential to note that there are various treatment options available for those with pelvic floor disorders.

Treatment options can range from lifestyle changes, such as dietary modifications and pelvic floor exercises, to more invasive procedures, such as surgery. Pelvic floor physical therapy is a popular treatment option that aims to improve pelvic floor function through exercises and stretches.

In some cases, medication may also be prescribed to help manage symptoms, such as pain and incontinence. Additionally, emotional support and counseling can help patients cope with the emotional and psychological impact of pelvic floor disorders.

What happens if you don't fix your pelvic floor?

Pelvic floor dysfunction (PFD) is a common condition that affects millions of people worldwide. It is estimated that more than 25% of women and 20% of men suffer from some form of PFD in their lifetime. PFD refers to a wide range of conditions that affect the muscles, ligaments, and tissues that support the pelvic organs, including the bladder, uterus, and rectum. These conditions can cause a variety of uncomfortable symptoms, such as urinary incontinence, fecal incontinence, painful intercourse, and pelvic pain. If left untreated, PFD can lead to a range of complications, so it's essential to seek medical attention if you experience any symptoms.

The pelvic floor is a group of muscles and ligaments that support the bladder, rectum, and uterus in women. It also helps control the urinary and bowel functions and sexual activity. PFD can occur when these muscles and ligaments weaken, resulting in a range of symptoms that can interfere with daily life.

If you don't fix your PFD, you can experience several complications. One of the most common complications is urinary tract infections (UTIs). UTIs occur when bacteria enter the urethra and travel up to the bladder, causing an infection. Women are more likely to develop UTIs than men, and PFD can increase the risk. When PFD weakens the pelvic floor muscles, it can cause the bladder to sag, leading to incomplete bladder emptying, which creates a favorable environment for bacteria growth.

Another potential complication of untreated PFD is fecal incontinence, which refers to the inability to control bowel movements. PFD can cause damage to the anal sphincter muscles, which can lead to bowel leakage. Fecal incontinence can be a very distressing and embarrassing problem that can significantly impact the quality of life.

Sexual dysfunction is another complication of untreated PFD. When the pelvic floor muscles are weak or damaged, it can cause painful intercourse or difficulty achieving orgasm. It can also lead to a decrease in sexual desire and self-esteem.

Untreated PFD can also lead to the development of pelvic organ prolapse (POP), a condition that occurs when the pelvic organs, such as the bladder or uterus, sag or fall out of place. POP can cause a bulge in the vagina, pain or pressure in the pelvis, and difficulty emptying the bladder or rectum. It can significantly impact a person's quality of life and require surgery to correct.

Chapter Ten

Living with a Pelvic Floor Disorder

Pelvic floor dysfunction is a condition that can cause a variety of symptoms, including urinary and fecal incontinence, pelvic pain, and sexual dysfunction. Living with a pelvic floor disorder can be challenging, both physically and emotionally. However, there are several strategies and treatments available that can help people manage their symptoms and improve their quality of life.

The first step in living with a pelvic floor disorder is to seek medical attention. A healthcare provider can perform a physical exam and diagnostic tests to determine the underlying cause of the symptoms. Depending on the diagnosis, the provider may recommend a variety of treatments, including medication, pelvic floor physical therapy, and surgery.

Pelvic floor physical therapy is often recommended as a first-line treatment for pelvic floor disorders. This type of therapy involves working with a trained physical therapist to learn exercises and techniques that can help strengthen and relax the pelvic floor muscles. These exercises may include Kegels, biofeedback, and manual therapy. In addition to physical therapy, lifestyle changes such as avoiding constipation, maintaining a healthy weight, and reducing stress can also be helpful in managing pelvic floor symptoms.

For some people, medication may be recommended to manage their symptoms. Medications may include muscle relaxants, anticholinergics, or antidepressants. Surgery may also be an option for those with severe symptoms that do not respond to other treatments.

In addition to medical treatments, there are also several strategies that can help people cope with the emotional impact of a pelvic floor disorder. One of the most important things is to talk openly with a healthcare provider or a mental health professional about the challenges and feelings associated with the condition. Joining a support group or online community of people who are going through similar experiences can also be helpful in reducing feelings of isolation and providing emotional support.

It is also important to take care of oneself physically and mentally. This may include engaging in regular exercise or physical activity, eating a healthy diet, getting enough sleep, and practicing stress-management techniques such as meditation or yoga.

Living with a pelvic floor disorder can be challenging, but it is important to remember that help is available. Seeking medical attention, participating in physical therapy, and making lifestyle changes can all be helpful in managing symptoms. Talking openly with healthcare providers and seeking emotional support can also be valuable in coping with the emotional impact of the condition. With the right treatment and support, people can live full and satisfying lives despite their pelvic floor disorder.

Chapter Eleven

Frequently Asked Questions

Pelvic floor dysfunction is a common condition that affects many people, particularly women. It can cause a variety of uncomfortable symptoms, such as incontinence, pelvic pain, and sexual dysfunction. As such, it is no surprise that many people have questions about this condition. Below we will explore some frequently asked questions about pelvic floor dysfunction and provide answers to help individuals better understand this condition.

What is pelvic floor dysfunction?

Pelvic floor dysfunction refers to a condition where the muscles and connective tissues of the pelvic floor are weak, tight, or dysfunctional. This can lead to a range of symptoms, including urinary or fecal incontinence, constipation, pain during sex, and chronic pelvic pain.

What causes pelvic floor dysfunction?

Pelvic floor dysfunction can be caused by a variety of factors, including childbirth, obesity, chronic constipation, certain medical conditions such as endometriosis, and even certain types of exercises. Some individuals may also have a genetic predisposition to this condition.

How is pelvic floor dysfunction diagnosed?

Pelvic floor dysfunction can be diagnosed through a physical exam by a healthcare provider who specializes in pelvic floor disorders. In some cases, diagnostic imaging tests, such as ultrasound or MRI, may also be necessary to determine the extent of the dysfunction.

What are the treatment options for pelvic floor dysfunction?

Treatment options for pelvic floor dysfunction can vary depending on the severity of the condition and the specific symptoms being experienced. Some common treatment options include pelvic floor physical therapy, medication, changes to diet and lifestyle, and surgery in more severe cases.

Can pelvic floor dysfunction be prevented?

In some cases, pelvic floor dysfunction can be prevented through lifestyle modifications, such as maintaining a healthy weight, practicing pelvic floor exercises, and avoiding certain exercises or activities that can strain the pelvic floor. Additionally, seeking treatment for medical conditions that can contribute to pelvic floor dysfunction, such as chronic constipation or endometriosis, can help prevent the development of this condition.

Is pelvic floor dysfunction a common condition?

Yes, pelvic floor dysfunction is a common condition that affects millions of people, particularly women. It is estimated that up to one-third of all women will experience some form of pelvic floor dysfunction in their lifetime.

Can pelvic floor dysfunction affect sexual function?

Yes, pelvic floor dysfunction can lead to sexual dysfunction, including pain during sex and difficulty achieving orgasm. This can have a significant impact on an individual's quality of life and should be addressed with a healthcare provider.

Can pelvic floor dysfunction be cured?

In many cases, pelvic floor dysfunction can be effectively treated or managed, allowing individuals to improve their symptoms and quality of life. However, in some cases, the condition may be chronic and require ongoing management.

What can I do to manage my pelvic floor dysfunction symptoms?

There are several things individuals can do to manage their pelvic floor dysfunction symptoms, including practicing pelvic floor exercises, maintaining a healthy diet and lifestyle, seeking treatment for any underlying medical conditions, and seeking support from a healthcare provider or support group.

Can men develop pelvic floor dysfunction?

Yes, while pelvic floor dysfunction is more commonly seen in women, men can also develop this condition. It is most commonly associated with chronic prostate issues or post-prostatectomy surgery.

Chapter Twelve

Quick tips

Pelvic floor health is essential for overall well-being, yet many people know little about how this complex group of muscles affects daily life. Whether you are experiencing symptoms, recovering from injury, or simply want to strengthen and maintain your pelvic floor, these practical tips will empower you with knowledge and actionable steps. Use these tips to better understand, care for, and treat pelvic floor disorders effectively.

- Learn the anatomy of your pelvic floor muscles to better understand their function
- Practice proper posture to reduce unnecessary pelvic floor strain
- Perform pelvic floor exercises (Kegels) regularly but avoid overdoing them
- Focus on correct technique when doing pelvic floor contractions
- Avoid holding your breath while exercising your pelvic floor
- Incorporate diaphragmatic breathing to support pelvic floor relaxation
- Use biofeedback devices if recommended to improve muscle

awareness

- Maintain a healthy weight to reduce pressure on your pelvic floor
- Stay hydrated but avoid excessive caffeine which can irritate the bladder
- Manage constipation to prevent added strain on pelvic muscles
- Eat a high-fiber diet to promote regular bowel movements
- Avoid heavy lifting or learn proper techniques to protect your pelvic floor
- Take frequent breaks if you have a sedentary job to move and stretch
- Try yoga or Pilates to strengthen core and pelvic muscles gently
- Avoid high-impact exercises if they worsen symptoms
- Consult a pelvic floor physiotherapist for personalized guidance
- Use warm baths or heat packs to relieve pelvic muscle tension
- Practice mindfulness or meditation to reduce pelvic floor tension caused by stress
- Avoid crossing your legs for long periods to maintain good pelvic alignment
- Learn to identify when your pelvic floor muscles are too tight or too weak
- Don't ignore urinary urgency or leakage symptoms—seek early

help

- Avoid constipation-causing medications if possible or discuss alternatives
- Practice bladder training techniques to improve control
- Avoid straining during bowel movements; take your time on the toilet
- Use a footstool to achieve a better posture when using the toilet
- Avoid prolonged sitting on hard surfaces to reduce pelvic pressure
- Wear comfortable, breathable clothing and underwear
- Avoid wearing tight pants that may restrict pelvic circulation
- Learn relaxation techniques to ease pelvic muscle spasms
- Track your symptoms in a diary to share with your healthcare provider
- Use pelvic floor muscle relaxation exercises if you experience pain or tightness
- Avoid high sugar diets that may worsen bladder symptoms
- Take pelvic floor breaks during long drives or flights
- Avoid smoking, as it can worsen coughing and pelvic floor strain
- Practice slow, controlled pelvic floor muscle releases after contraction
- Use a mirror or smartphone camera to check your pelvic floor

exercise form

- Avoid jumping or running on hard surfaces if you have pelvic pain
- Gradually increase exercise intensity to avoid muscle fatigue
- Include strength training for core muscles along with pelvic floor work
- Avoid bearing down during pelvic floor exercises
- Use breathing to assist with pelvic floor relaxation during exercises
- Avoid prolonged periods of coughing or seek treatment for chronic cough
- Schedule regular pelvic floor assessments if you have risk factors
- Be patient; pelvic floor recovery can take weeks or months
- Use vaginal weights or cones if prescribed to build muscle strength
- Avoid excessive use of pads or liners to prevent skin irritation
- Maintain good hygiene to avoid infections that can irritate the pelvic floor
- Incorporate pelvic floor stretches into your daily routine
- Avoid jumping to conclusions—get a proper diagnosis for pelvic symptoms
- Don't self-diagnose; consult a healthcare professional for tailored advice
- Use warm compresses to soothe pelvic floor muscle cramps

- Include hip and lower back stretches to support pelvic alignment
- Avoid tight diaphragmatic muscles that can cause pelvic floor dysfunction
- Practice good ergonomics at your workstation to support pelvic health
- Avoid high heels for long periods which may alter pelvic posture
- Track fluid intake to balance hydration and bladder health
- Learn proper breathing patterns during physical activity
- Avoid constipation by not ignoring the urge to defecate
- Use relaxation apps or guided imagery to reduce pelvic tension
- Explore pelvic floor physical therapy exercises customized to your needs
- Use gentle massage techniques to relieve pelvic muscle knots
- Avoid carrying heavy bags on one side to prevent pelvic imbalance
- Stay consistent with your pelvic floor exercise routine
- Avoid overstretching pelvic muscles to prevent instability
- Try aquatic therapy if land exercises cause discomfort
- Learn about the connection between pelvic floor and sexual health
- Avoid excessive alcohol which can irritate bladder function

- Use bladder diaries to monitor frequency and fluid intake
- Be aware of your pelvic floor during everyday activities like coughing or sneezing
- Avoid holding urine for long periods to prevent bladder issues
- Practice correct toilet posture to reduce pelvic strain
- Include relaxation breaks during busy days to prevent pelvic tension
- Avoid excessive use of laxatives without medical advice
- Explore mindfulness-based stress reduction for chronic pelvic pain
- Avoid harsh soaps or products around the pelvic area
- Learn about the effects of pregnancy and childbirth on pelvic floor health
- Use support garments if recommended during postpartum recovery
- Avoid ignoring signs of pelvic organ prolapse
- Engage in low-impact aerobic activities to maintain overall fitness
- Avoid excessive repetitive movements that strain the pelvis
- Consult a dietitian if dietary changes are needed for bowel health
- Learn pelvic floor muscle coordination exercises
- Practice abdominal bracing combined with pelvic floor activation

- Avoid excessive use of tampons if experiencing pelvic discomfort
- Maintain open communication with your healthcare providers
- Avoid prolonged bed rest which can weaken pelvic muscles
- Try transcutaneous electrical nerve stimulation (TENS) for pain relief if advised
- Avoid self-massage without guidance to prevent injury
- Learn to relax the pelvic floor during sexual activity for comfort
- Avoid tight pelvic muscles caused by stress or anxiety
- Practice slow and controlled breathing to ease muscle tension
- Use pillows to support pelvic positioning during rest
- Avoid excessive consumption of bladder irritants like citrus or spicy foods
- Learn safe ways to resume exercise after pelvic surgery or childbirth
- Avoid heavy lifting immediately postpartum
- Monitor menstrual cycle changes that may affect pelvic symptoms
- Include partner support and education for pelvic floor disorders
- Use pelvic floor training apps to guide exercises
- Avoid excessive pelvic floor contractions which can cause muscle fatigue

- Recognize when symptoms need urgent medical attention
- Learn the difference between pelvic floor relaxation and strengthening exercises
- Practice pelvic floor exercises in different positions to find what works best
- Avoid delaying treatment for pelvic floor symptoms to prevent worsening
- Incorporate relaxation techniques before bedtime to reduce pelvic tension
- Use warm showers to relax pelvic muscles
- Avoid overly aggressive physical therapy techniques without professional supervision

Have Questions / Comments?

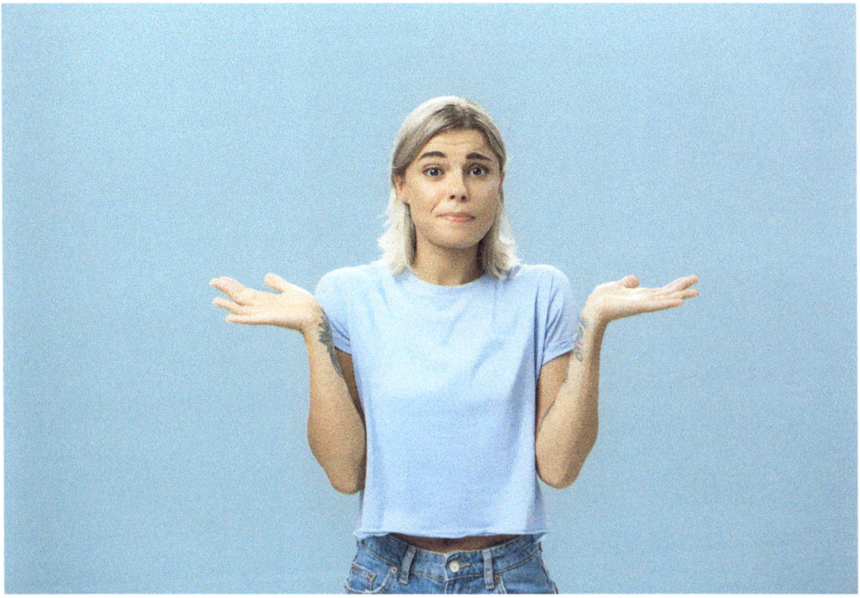

This book was designed to cover as much information as possible, but I know I have probably missed something, or some new amazing discovery has just come out.

If you notice something missing or have a question that I failed to answer, please get in touch and let me know. If I can, I will email you an answer and also update the book so others can also benefit from it.

Thanks For Being Awesome :)

Submit Your Questions / Comments At:

https://questions.xspurts.com

Get Free Stuff

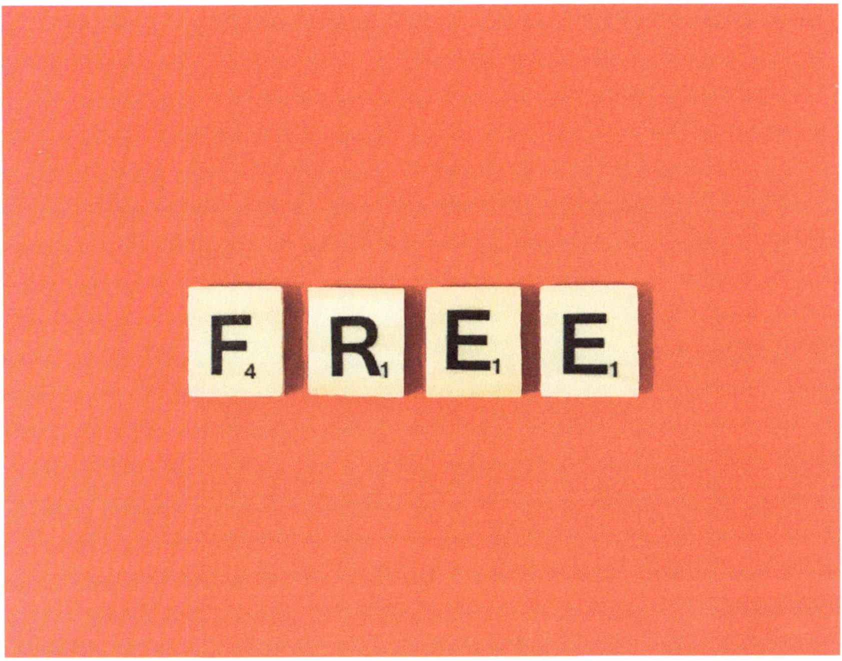

We love writing and have produced a huge number of books.

For being one of our amazing readers, we would love to offer you more books we have created, 100% free.

To claim this limited time special offer, simply go to the site below and enter your name and email address.

You will then receive loads (as we love our readers so much :) of our great books, content and audio direct to your email account, 100% free!

Get Loads of FREE Stuff at:

https://free.xspurts.com

* 9 7 8 1 7 7 6 8 4 6 9 8 6 *
SD - #0196 - 070926 - C0 - 229/152/8 - PB - 9781776846986 - Matt Lamination